THE
SECRET ART
OF
BOABOM

Also by Asanaro

The Secret Art of Seamm-Jasani

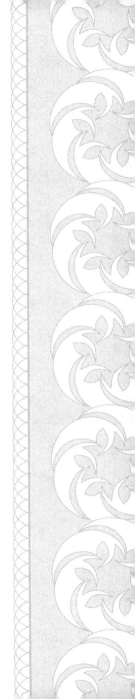

Jeremy P. Tarcher / Penguin
a member of Penguin Group (USA) Inc.

2006
In the year of the Emenise

THE
SECRET ART
OF
BOABOM

• • • •

Awaken Inner Power Through
Defense-Meditation from Ancient Tibet

ASANARO

TRANSLATED BY JOICE BUCCAREY

ILLUSTRATED BY ASANARO

EDITED BY BENJAMIN B. KELLEY

JEREMY P. TARCHER / PENGUIN
Published by the Penguin Group

Penguin Group (USA) Inc., 375 Hudson Street, New York, New York 10014, USA · Penguin Group (Canada), 90 Eglinton Avenue East, Suite 700, Toronto, Ontario M4P 2Y3, Canada (a division of Pearson Penguin Canada Inc.) · Penguin Books Ltd, 80 Strand, London WC2R 0RL, England · Penguin Ireland, 25 St Stephen's Green, Dublin 2, Ireland (a division of Penguin Books Ltd) · Penguin Group (Australia), 250 Camberwell Road, Camberwell, Victoria 3124, Australia (a division of Pearson Australia Group Pty Ltd) · Penguin Books India Pvt Ltd, 11 Community Centre, Panchsheel Park, New Delhi–110 017, India · Penguin Group (NZ), Cnr Airborne and Rosedale Roads, Albany, Auckland 1310, New Zealand (a division of Pearson New Zealand Ltd) · Penguin Books (South Africa) (Pty) Ltd, 24 Sturdee Avenue, Rosebank, Johannesburg 2196, South Africa

Penguin Books Ltd, Registered Offices: 80 Strand, London WC2R 0RL, England

Library of Congress Cataloging-in-Publication Data

Asanaro, date.
    The secret art of boabom : awaken inner power through defense-meditation from ancient Tibet / Asanaro ; translated by Joice Buccarey; illustrated by Asanaro ; edited by Benjamin B. Kelley.
        p.   cm.
    ISBN 1-58542-521-4
    1. Self-care, Health—China—Tibet. 2. Medicine, Tibetan. 3. Exercise—China—Tibet. I. Title.
RA776.95.A83   2006   2006045631
613—dc22

Book design by Lovedog Studio

Neither the publisher nor the author is engaged in rendering professional advice or services to the individual reader. The ideas, procedures, and suggestions contained in this book are not intended as a substitute for consulting with your physician. All matters regarding your health require medical supervision. Neither the author nor the publisher shall be liable or responsible for any loss or damage allegedly arising from any information or suggestion in this book.

While the author has made every effort to provide accurate telephone numbers and Internet addresses at the time of publication, neither the publisher nor the author assumes any responsibility for errors, or for changes that occur after publication. Further, the publisher does not have any control over and does not assume any responsibility for author or third-party websites or their content.

146119709

To the Boabom Arts.
To the Guides and Apprentices who were,
who are, and who shall come.

CONTENTS

The Steps of Boabom

. . .

. . .

THE
SECRET ART
OF
BOABOM

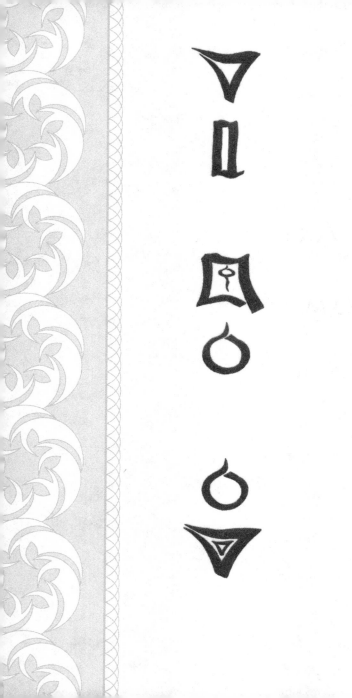

Not knowing a Guide
is like a Temple
without its sacred writings to direct it.

Not knowing the Way
is like a Temple
immersed in corruption.

Not knowing a Lover
is like a Temple
with no divinity to adore.

Not knowing the Mind
is like a Temple
built for an unknown reason.

Not knowing the Art
is like a Temple
whose members are weak and impressionable.

Not knowing the righteousness of one's own Body
is like a Temple
abandoned to Chaos.

—*from* The Memories of the Mmulargan

THE STEPS OF BOABOM

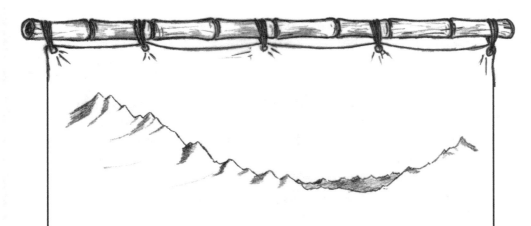

INTRODUCTION

T HE ROOTS of Boabom are lost in time. Its origin is in ancient
Tibet, several thousand years before the birth of the Buddha, before the Vedas were written, and before the Chinese Empire even
thought to exist. Even though we cannot say about that era that nations or countries existed as we know nations and countries to exist
today, we can say that the land of the Himalayas and the high plateau
were always a flourishing field for encounters of different cultures
and mixtures of races and clans. Among them was one that left a
silent inheritance to us, and the time has now come to share it.

The teaching of Boabom is distinguished by its broadminded-
ness, its depth, and its positive way of looking at life, as well as the
consubstantial harmonic relationship that must exist between body
and mind, without the restriction and prejudice that religions would
later dictate. As such, its Arts are not limited to a certain type of

. . .

movement or to intricate metaphysical theories; instead their range is practical, from relaxation, breathing, and meditation to defense, dance, philosophy, and much more, with its sole objective to make "this life" an Art in itself.

I am certain that all of this must come as a surprise to many, mainly those who limit the existence of Tibet to the country of the Buddhist tradition, or to yoga, while relegating any exercise concerning relaxation or forms of defense exclusively to India, China, or the other Eastern countries. This is not so, and there is still much to be discovered and learned from the Land of Snows, despite those who will not be happy to recognize this fact.

Tibet's valleys and secluded landscapes still hold surprises and stories yet untold. It was one of these surprises I met with many years ago: Boabom. This teaching has always been a pilgrim's secret, and those who migrated to transmit this Way continued to prefer that secrecy over great publicity. What I was given as a consequence of this pilgrimage was given in silence; in that way it was developed and valued, in the quietness of privacy and in the productive and irreproducible dialogue between Guide and Apprentice. I could never even intend to transmit this experience fully, for it is something very personal, yet I do want this book to be a candle for many who search, as I did, for the elusive balance between the body and the mind, with its hidden abilities.

A few years ago, moved by unpredictable circumstances, I wrote the book *The Secret Art of Seamm-Jasani*, an introduction to a system corresponding to a kind of "gentle" Boabom. The warm reception that book received showed that there are many who seek something beyond what is trumpeted by the media. In the wake of its success, it was natural that I should show the other face of this teaching: developed here, in the work you now hold in your hands.

This book describes Boabom, considered an Art of Defense. However, in order to understand it, readers and students need feel the word "defense" not as such, but from a new perspective that goes beyond the everyday to relate to energy and self-awareness, and therefore to meditation and internal balance.

In order that this may be understood in the correct way, I have composed this book from three perspectives, which, in one way or another, are knitted together and will satisfy all readers at their own measure.

The First Step of this work is a tale that introduces the intellectual student to the transcendental ideas of this teaching, to its "thoughts," its forms for seeing life, while at the same time it is a detailed explanation of Boabom itself. This story represents the *Mind* of the Art and is also linked to the book on Seamm-Jasani, as well as books to come in the future.

The Second Step describes Boabom itself. This point is made for the restless student who wants to experience the meditative-defensive technique in practice, to sweat and feel its benefits and effects, and through this to understand the story told in the first part. This Step can be seen as an introductory course for beginning students. In it you will see that everyone can learn this system, without any prior knowledge. This Step, as the development of the practical part or the method, represents the *Art* itself.

Finally, the Third Step is dedicated to the practical reader who likes knowing with certainty the ground on which she or he is stepping. This section deals with the School itself through its students, who speak of their own real and daily experience. It also includes the first scientific study made of Boabom, which details the practical results of this teaching from the perspective of both modern medicine and psychology. This last section represents the *Body* of the Art, our need to grow roots and walk with our feet on the ground in order to allow our internal vision to quietly contemplate the universe.

Today the Boabom Art continues its own life, as does its School, existing disconnected from any cultural or national attachment. Boabom lives in its students and its teachers, and in the energy of search and transmission that they will continue to generate in the dream of the future. May the stellar winds blow favorably to all of them, and especially to you!

Welcome to Boabom, the Art of the Great Plateau!

Asanaro
In the year of the Emenise

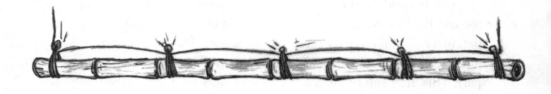

First Step

THE WAY

Chapter 1

GUIDE AND APPRENTICE

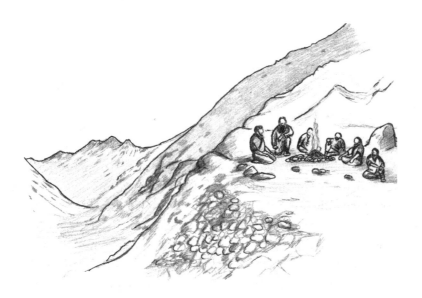

Wisdom is not enlarged by the number. . . .

—Alsam, from The Secret Art of Seamm-Jasani

FIRE HAS THAT strange capacity of seduction, of dancing with the thoughts. . . .

With that subtle power it presented itself before a wandering group in the secluded mountain valleys . . . on the roof of the world or perhaps at the end of it—where is not important.

The flames flowed gently upward, plasma of movement, symbol of the ineffable dance of life and magic.

One of those passengers through the loneliness, one Apprentice in particular was sinking into a nighttime vision of his own, buoyed only by the resplendent flame reflected in the faces of all those who surrounded that light, watching in silence.

The night was plentiful with stars, silent guides, messengers of an indecipherable language. The sky showed the Great Way in all its splendor. Meanwhile the bonfire, protected by a measured, careful circle of stones, projected its volatile sparks like little seeds, thrown to the heights, seeking a fertile field in which to nestle and to turn, at the auspicious moment, into stars themselves, into bright stars that would drive the steps of the pilgrims who will come in the dream of the future.

The small group kept a respectful silence, waiting for the precious words of their Guide. He was the eldest among them, and he sat, strangely silent, within himself secretly recalling his own stories and time as an apprentice. He watched those who followed him and somehow saw himself, his own curiosities and mistakes, the longings and illusions of his youth. His eyes shone in the light of the bonfire, more so even than the eyes of those who wished to learn from him, who in those moments wanted to capture some of his vitality, catch his thoughts, uncover his secrets. The younger ones were watching him, wondering what it was that set him so apart from all rules, wondering where his eternal smile came from, or his inexhaustible energy, strength, and restlessness. What was his source? Was he born with it? Had he learned it somewhere? Is it born from cultivating the Arts of which they were students? Could they grab hold of the aura that surrounded him? Could they catch the ghost of strength that was always by his side?

The restless Apprentice continued to observe, from the fire to the eyes of his Guide. He had many questions within him, but he did not want to interrupt that moment. There are only a few moments like that one, and when they occur, the precise words or suitable questions that could dare to interrupt such silence are always hard to find. He preferred the silence anyway: after all, there had been a great activity since dawn.

It had been early when the small group of students awoke to their duties and lessons in the Gentle Art; more, even, for in the afternoon their lessons had continued. Just at dusk it had been time for Boabom, the Osseous Art, born with the stars, the mysterious, lonely mystic, the precious jewel in the hands of the wise man who knows how to value and polish it. After the lesson of the morning and the lesson that was born with the setting of the great star, all there deserved a great rest.

Despite the incongruousness of questions in that moment, one of the newest students in the group, staring, beardless and curious, dared to break the silence. With a tone of innocence, he asked a question.

"Guide . . ." He spoke with a bit of hesitation. "I have been following your teaching and Art for a while now, but I'd like to ask you something. It may seem silly after all that I've learned, but . . . what really is the Boabom Art?"

The thoughtful teacher kept his silence for a moment. Smiling, he touched his long beard, which was already showing one or two gray hairs, and without answering he addressed the restless Apprentice, who was sitting just beside the young man who had asked the question. He only said:

"Tell me, Black Sheep . . . how would you answer that question?"

He was a bit surprised to hear the Guide so directly inviting him to offer a solution to the younger one's question. He was even more surprised that the Guide had called him thusly, for the Guide had only just begun to call him that in the morning. He wasn't sure if he had been given that name as a positive symbol of his character in the Art or because of his way, a little irascible and rebellious. Yet once he had recovered from this surprise, he answered.

"I do not know . . . I think you are the right person to answer that, and I would feel as if I were overstepping myself if I did."

The Guide replied very directly. "You are the apprentice who has been with me the longest, who has begun teaching as well as learning, and if you feel ready for that, you probably have something to say."

Black Sheep did not know if the Guide's words were a reproach or an approval. However, he now had to answer; for after all, it was true that he had begun helping out with the classes a while ago, and that he was already beginning to have his own students. Maybe with time he would want to teach many more than was normal in this Art, and these intentions knit in his mind had been easily read by his Guide; this seemed one of the reasons for his new nickname. The Apprentice tried to base his words on what he had heard from his mentor as well as on what he felt, himself, and after a few moments finally answered.

"Well . . . it's a simple, concrete question, ideal for a direct answer." The flames of the central fire grew as he continued, more confident in his explanation. "All of us, when we begin, may have seen Boabom as an Art of Relaxation, or perhaps as a strange Art of Defense, but in some way or another it has surprised us all, for Boabom has a thousand ways, just as it has a thousand movements. Each of them is a thread that is woven into a great fabric, which seen up close reveals only individual threads. If we want to know its real shape, we must take some distance and gain a wider view that will allow us to discover its real features." He continued without pause, inspired by the bonfire, the loneliness of the mountains, and the stars above. "To me, the Art is poetry, legend, life, and these transform it into a restless internal spark. I think of a phrase I have heard in my lessons: 'The visible threads of Boabom are the shapes of its movements, but the reality can only be observed by each, in his own experience.'"

There was a pause, and the Guide spoke. "Good, Black Sheep," and he added, addressing the rest of the students, "Which one of you would like to add something to what he has said?"

One of them, tall and thin, replied. "Well, I would say that, just as our teaching has its relaxed, or gentle, face, Seamm-Jasani, it has the strong and fast face of Boabom. This one, more than just an Art of Defense, represents a channel of strength and energy that clears and feeds the mind in a direct, solid, uninhibited way. That is how I feel it myself."

The Guide took his time.

"Watch the fire, apprentices. What in it is so appealing? What fascinates and at the same time calms us so?"

Another of the young faces answered, trying the correct answer. "Its heat?"

Another followed. "Its red and yellow colors that change?"

Again the guide spoke. "Each of these elements is correct, but what inevitably attracts us is its movement. Its movement, generating waves that trespass our senses and feed our mind, our interior world, reflecting and reacting continuously in movement. Boabom is a dance projected as a precise, unique, and extraordinary form of energy that to common eyes seems a defense as subtle as unexpected, yet which goes far beyond. Few will be able to see, for few are prepared to seriously deepen their paths and dare to discover the ultimate end: what is hidden within. Many can clamor to the door of the Art, which is crowded with enthusiasts, and yet so few reach its central chamber: there you will find but a few guests."

The students were becoming more enthusiastic, with the night and the words of their teacher, and little by little they dared to ask more questions.

One of them spoke quickly. "But what is the 'door of the Art'? And what is its 'central chamber'?"

The Guide, not wishing to answer, simply gazed sideways at Black Sheep, who answered in his stead.

"I think, by your example, you mean that the 'door' is the external face of its teaching, what most people see and can relate quickly to what they already know, to all of their preconceived ideas. So I think that the door of the Art is when we see it as a form of defense, as simply another technique, and we are unable to venture into its depths. That is why its entrance is full of people. As with everything, no one wants or really cares about going deeper, to discover what is really there, for that requires sacrifice, effort, and discipline."

"Good point," answered the Guide, as he opened up another question. "But what would its 'central chamber' be?"

The students were silent; no one dared to give a more assertive answer, not even the oldest apprentice.

One of them only said, "And you, Guide, could you give us an answer, so we can understand that example?"

"Yes, I could," he answered as he began quietly to prod the fire. They all seemed to prick up their ears in expectation of an answer, but none came. After a moment, he added quietly, "Or I could tell you a story, and you could come to your own conclusions."

No one said a word; they just looked at each other, all silently thinking that perhaps if they chose the story they would miss the answer, or that if they chose the answer he could choose simply not to answer and they would miss the story. After all, their Guide was everything but predictable and open about the teachings; there were only a few times like that night, when they could get at some of his knowledge. Besides, it was always after a huge effort, after showing a huge devotion to the Art that they were able to learn a lesson from him. After having known him for a while, it was clear to all of them that he felt that if none of them deserved it, he would rather die and take all the deepest secrets of his teachings to the grave and oblivion.

One of them finally broke the silence. "Tell us the story, then. It is much better for each of us to find our own ideas in it." And they all looked at one another, seeming to approve of what the student was saying. The Black Sheep was silent.

The Guide continued his ministrations with the fire for a few moments. Then he added new logs, and the bonfire grew stronger. The air from the mountains has always been cold, even more so on clear nights such as this one, and the heat was welcome to the whole group. They could feel the heat on their faces, in contrast to the chilly breeze off the cliffs. They all remained silent, wanting the story to begin.

"All right. Tonight seems to favor a good story: it will suit some of you. Pay attention to the details, and you will learn some more about the Art of which you are students."

Again they smiled at each other, surprised at the opportunity they were being given, for it was quite uncommon for their Guide to tell them a story about Boabom. They made themselves as comfortable as they could.

The night shone its finest stars, and in that moment each of the students anxiously awaited the words of their Guide, all trying to concentrate as best they could on what they were about to hear, and hopeful that if they were able to, they would understand the profound meaning of the Boabom Art, the depths of its movements and appearance.

They held a respectful silence, trying to forget their daily concerns, the towns and villages from which they came and the work that awaited them there.

Together with the silence from the skies and the gentle song of the breeze from the heights, the story began. . . .

Chapter 2

THE WANDERER

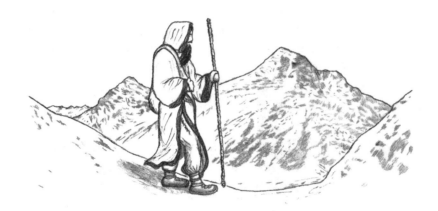

*When the Apprentice is ready,
the Guide will come.*

—*traditional proverb*

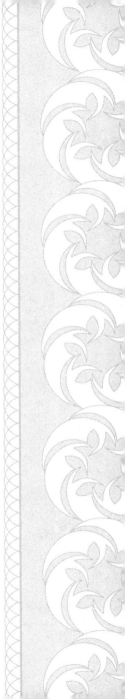

WHAT I AM about to tell you can be traced back many centuries into the past, to ancient mountains and valleys filled with legends and hidden tales, hidden even more for those who are not able to see the details! In this time, long past, wars and battles were common amongst the villages." After smiling to himself, he continued. "Well, that is something that has not changed so much. Let's just say that it was a time when the conflicts were more audacious and less organized than they are today.

"In one of these faraway mountain villages lived the hero of our tale: a graceful young lady, daughter of a hardworking peasant family. Her parents had named her Tara, and for them life was their seven children, their land, their animals, and, of course, their gods.

"The childhood of our girl was quiet and without great beginnings, spent amongst playing and daily duties. As with every good young woman, she was prepared in the work allotted her gender: caring for her four older brothers, caring for her two younger sisters, while cooking, cleaning the house, and mending the family's clothing. Of course, as she grew older, her mother used Tara's spare time to teach her how to make herself pretty, and though the girl cared little for this, being perhaps a task too much belonging to her gender, in order to avoid any arguments with her mother and sisters, the girl learned, albeit with resignation.

"On the other side, her brothers were becoming experts in horseback riding, arrogantly displaying their skills before the town girls. From time to time, they would display their battlefield skills, something that the men of those villages were famous for. Tara only watched.

"Years passed, and little by little the girl became a woman. The problem was that somehow she did not fit in with what was around her. Young women her age spoke only about marriage and children, while she fantasized alone of faraway places and valleys she had never seen. And without telling anyone, she traveled in her dreams.

"In those years a large conflict grew in the borderlands near their village." The storyteller paused as he continued to feed the fire that lit the faces of the curious apprentices. In that moment, the youngest of them again dared to interrupt the story.

"But Guide, what country was it, and whom were they fighting against? Was it a big fight? Were the people from the village in the right?"

All the rest gazed seriously at him, since none wanted to interrupt, yet many of them were asking themselves the very same questions.

The Guide answered: "You must know that when it comes to a war—no matter where it comes from, no matter where it is produced, who effects it more or who benefits from it—war is always a looting in which, sooner or later, everyone is a victim, while a few are astute . . . well . . . executioners. So do not worry about the name of the country of this story. It is irrelevant."

Another of the students spoke right away and said, almost apologizing for the other student's interruption: "Please, continue. We want to know what happened."

The Guide became comfortable again and gazing still into the fire continued.

"Well, as I was saying, the war grew quickly, and the conflicts came to the village. Almost all of the men took their horses and went off to the fight with enthusiasm; they could finally show what great fighters and 'men' they were. Unable to do anything to stop them, the girl watched as her father and older brothers left. To the fortune of the village, as well as of the women, who had been left in charge of everything, the conflict never reached the town itself. Yet they still suffered the consequences. Men began to return, injured and frustrated at seeing themselves stuck in a war with no results. Most died in battles and skirmishes, but worse off were those who survived, who had the marks of those battles tattooed like indelible scars into their minds. Tara's four brothers died in combat; only her father returned. He changed much after that loss: he grew sullen and irascible, drowning his sorrow in fermented drinks. Her mother became quiet and sad. Only daughters remained in the family, and parents without sons had little to be proud of in those times and places.

"Both of Tara's younger sisters affected a good disposition toward their miserable father, but as soon as he was no longer watching, they burst out, no longer hiding their increasing disdain toward him, as well as his constant railing against women.

"Tara, meanwhile, remained silent, trying to calm herself and to calm them all, yet she felt the situation turning from bad to worse. She felt great compassion toward her father and even more toward her mother and sisters, even though they were always complaining about her silence.

"Alone, she continued to dream, feeling that everything could be different, that maybe the whole situation could change. She could always be seen gazing off at the horizon, looking at or waiting for no one knew what.

"To make matters worse, that season the crops were bad. The carelessness the war had brought was reaping its consequences. Most of the cattle were lost or given in compensation to the arrogance of the victors.

"Bit by bit, her father began drinking more and more. Nothing improved; everything turned worse. The family clearly felt that, in a way, he wished they had died instead of his sons. Sometimes, when he was angry, he would start to yell at them. 'You don't know how to ride a horse! You don't know how to fight! You're only a bunch of useless, weak women, not like my sons! What am I going to do with you? You can't even work a whole month! Who will fight for us? Who will bring back our cattle?' As the insults increased, a feeling of anger and impotence began to grow within Tara. She wished in those moments that she was a warrior able to defend her land, to show her father what she was really capable of doing. It seemed, however, that none of her dreams would come true.

"The snowy season began with the barns barely provisioned. But the cold and winds fanned by the mountains did not come alone that winter. Something out of the ordinary happened. . . .

"An older pilgrim, quiet and with a long gray beard, passed through the village, resting there for a few days and paying to stay in one of the nearby homes.

"Quickly the rumors ran through the village, though it was not the presence of a foreigner that called the attention of the people. Some said that he was surely following the route that all the pilgrims followed toward the sacred places, or that perhaps he was going to visit some relatives. The only thing that really surprised anyone was his accent; this was how they knew he was not from the nearby lands. Nevertheless, he was a kind and composed man. Many began calling him The Wanderer.

"Tara felt strangely curious about the visitor. Not able to help herself, she broke her father's rules and, leaving her work in the fields early one afternoon, went to go and meet the pilgrim. She had only to pay a visit to the neighbors who were housing him, which would be a fine excuse; besides, they were relatives of her mother. This, however, proved not to be enough, for whenever she went, he was not there. The woman of the house said that he was a very reserved man, that he rarely ate with them, and that because the winter had already closed the mountain passes, he had asked to stay the whole season in the little cabin just next to the house. He had also asked if he could pay for the use of a small, abandoned animal barn that belonged to the family and was half an hour walking toward the hills.

"She continued to persevere with her visits, moved by an instinct she could not explain. On one of these occasions, she simply followed one of the paths, which led to a plateau near the house where the man was staying. She thought perhaps she could find some wood for the winter near there, and that maybe she could meet the mysterious pilgrim and discover what he was doing in the shack he had rented.

"She walked in silence up the road. After a while she heard strange sounds; instinctively she tried not to make any noise. She hid behind one of the rocks and peeked over. What she saw left her in amazement.

"On a small plateau in front of the shack, the old man was moving like someone young and full of life. He no longer looked old in fact, nor did his beard seem so white in contrast with the mountain snows. His hands took graceful forms, moving with skill and harmony. At the same time, his steps were soft and confident, then in an instant fast and sharp. After every movement he made strange sounds, long and short, united with the sound of breathing and movement.

"She was fascinated, for she had never seen a dance of that kind, or anyone who moved in that way, with so much grace, skill, and confidence. He seemed so far from everything, so absorbed, so distant from the thoughts that distracted the peasants.

"She had heard stories from her uncles and other relatives, tales of legendary warriors, men who could accomplish great exploits, but she had never seen one of them up close, someone who was real, not just a cocky peasant. Was that strange man a real warrior, one whom the legends spoke about?

"She watched him for only an instant, and almost at the same time the man stopped his strange practices and made a gracious gesture, joining his hands in a very peculiar way. She became a little frightened and left the place quickly, without making any noise.

"The days passed, the winter grew colder, and the young woman continued to go in the afternoon to that same spot, to watch the strange wanderer of the mountains. She enjoyed observing his practices. Fearing he would forbid her from watching, she said nothing, trying instead to keep from being discovered. Later, secretly, she clumsily tried to imitate his movements, but she felt that she had neither the grace nor the agility she needed. But she did not let this discourage her. On one occasion, she went to the house where he was staying and brought an enormous piece of cheese as a present for the family, and, against all formalities, she brought a big piece for him. On that day she would finally see him face to face.

"He greeted her kindly but was mostly trivial in his conversation. They spoke a little about the weather, the region, and the local foods. Nevertheless, though she did not know why, she sensed that he observed her manners and behavior in detail. The woman of the house, who spoke with them, insisted on asking him what village he came from, but he gently avoided the subject. They only knew his name: Nnu-Suto.

"After a few moments he thanked her for the present and left. The woman and her husband remained, speaking with Tara about the visitor. On the one hand, they liked him, for he paid well, but, on the other hand, they did not, for he seemed strange. Besides, it was suspicious that he never made reference to the gods.

"The young woman did her best to finish the conversation quickly, and then quietly walked after the visitor: She knew that at that hour he would go to the same place to do his strange rituals. Silently she hid behind the same rocks to watch: The man was quiet, cleaning the space a little and moving some stones, as if preparing for his practices. At one moment in this, when he had his back turned to Tara and she was sure he had not discovered her, he spoke: "'Tara . . . that's what they call you, correct? Are you not bored with always spying on me?'

"She felt her heart jump up and come out of her mouth; for a few seconds she was totally mute. A terrible fear then came over her, for if her father discovered her actions, she would suffer all of his rage. Slowly she raised herself to standing and, in a halting, stuttering voice answered:

"'I . . . I am sorry, sir . . . it hasn't been my intention to interrupt or disturb you. I have been very imprudent.'

"He came a little closer and continued. 'Then what has your intention been for all of these days?'

"She became red with embarrassment, for it was obvious that he had noticed her presence from the very beginning. She stuttered again but answered spontaneously. 'What you do . . . deeply caught my attention. Are you a warrior?'

"He answered quietly. 'A warrior is only a servant of a master of war. I am neither a servant nor a master.'

"'But I have heard that there are warriors who make great exploits with their bodies . . . that is what you do?'

"The man said, laughing, 'Hahaha . . . being alive is a great exploit, young lady! Do not try to understand what I do . . . you will not come to the right conclusions.'

"She lowered her gaze and, calling strength from within herself, asked something she never believed she could. 'Could I learn what you do? Would you teach me?'

"The man laughed out loud, and said: 'Hahaha! What do you think this man can teach you? What do you think you can accomplish?'

"'I know you can teach me how to become a great warrior!' Then she added, doubtful, 'I know I am just a woman, but I am certain I can learn how to fight, and that you can show me how!'

"The man sat down on a nearby rock, so as not to fall over as he continued laughing. She felt belittled. He soon added: 'Why should I teach you? You are not prepared to learn; besides, you are only a woman. Give me a reason to teach you.'

"Her eyes filled with tears as he answered her in that way. It crossed her mind that, somehow, this was the same as what her father always told her: that she was only a woman. However, there was something different in this man's tone, something that made her think that he only wanted to infuriate her, and make her leave. She insisted: 'I know you liked my cheese. . . . Let me provide you with cheese, milk, and dried meat for the winter, and you can teach me!'

" 'That does not seem to be a good enough reason to teach you.' He then added, in a harsh tone, while watching to see her reaction, 'And besides . . . you will still only be a woman.'

"She lowered her head again, and again insisted. 'Teach me and you will see what I can learn.' She continued, smiling, 'Anyway, if you are a good teacher, you will make a good student of me, whether I am a woman or not.'

"The man laughed aloud again. He liked her energy and decisiveness, and he finally agreed but not without placing some conditions that, one way or another, he thought the girl would not be able to fulfill. She listened, attentive and enthusiastic.

" 'All right. I will accept you, but you must satisfy my conditions, which are the following: First, you will come here for your lesson every two days in the afternoon. After the second lesson you will rest for two days in a row, and on the third we will continue, and so on. If you miss a lesson, I will not teach you again. Second, you will be as punctual as you shall be constant, or you will not see me again. Third, you will come in comfortable clothes, fit for movement, not with that whole lot of skirts you are wearing now. Fourth, three or four hours before the lesson you will not eat heavy meals, but shortly after each lesson you will be able to eat whatever you want. Fifth, whatever I teach you is meant only for you, and if you show it, teach it, or use it in any way, I will not teach you again. Sixth, you will provide me with food every three days . . . this is enough for me,' and he added, looking carefully at her, 'As for the seventh point, you shall ask your father and mother for an authorization.' This sounded like a death sentence to the ears of Tara. He continued speaking, 'And eighth, you shall not argue about my teachings or the related conditions. If you can realize all of these points and agree to follow them without exception, I will await you here on the day after tomorrow.

"She replied, weakly, 'But . . .' The pilgrim interrupted her immediately. 'No buts . . . It is all or nothing.'

"Tara felt at this point that the number seven would be impossible to fulfill, and insisted, hoping he would free her from it.

"'I am old enough! I don't need either my father's or my mother's authorization to get married.'

"'You are already arguing with me . . . mmm . . . remember point eight,' he answered, smiling, and then added sharply, 'Besides, if you have been convincing enough to get me to teach you, you will easily convince them to allow you to take my lessons.'

"She nodded humbly, without any more complaining, for there was no other possibility. She agreed, and started thinking of how she was going to get their permission. Finally, she offered one last comment, a question: 'I will do as you ask, but I would like only to ask . . . if you could tell me . . . what is the name of your teaching?'

"He answered precisely: 'Boabom!'

"With the sound of this word the conversation was finished, and she left, happy but worried at the same time. She did not know how her family would react before the demand for their approval, especially since no one knew that wanderer or had any reference of him, his origin, or the origin of his Art."

Chapter 3

THE CLAN OF THE LONELY

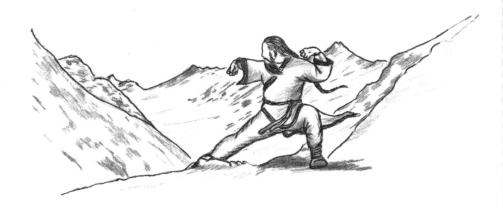

Who having authority to say "This is, this is not . . ."
if all of us through the day getting light from the same star,
and through the night getting light from the same moon?

—Omboni, *"The Memotecarian,"*
from The Legend of the Mmulmmat

THE NEXT DAY Tara silently prepared the food she had promised, leaving it in the cabin that served as a house for the mysterious wanderer, though she still did not have the agreed upon permission. Better said, she had not dared ask for it. Finally, the evening before the day of the first lesson, she gathered the courage to ask her parents; she was terribly afraid of being chastised for her curiosity and desire to learn from the foreigner. She could just imagine what her father would say. "Women! Always snooping around and causing trouble. Why aren't my sons alive?" She was not afraid of the yelling, but what really worried her was that, in the end, he or her mother could refuse her request and thus she would lose this opportunity to learn what, to her eyes, seemed such a strange warrior's dance.

It seemed, however, that the winds were blowing in her favor, for everything was quiet when she returned home from working in the fields. A short while later her father walked in through the main door. He was unusually kind to her, for it seemed that, after all, he felt that she was the only one who still had real feelings for him, unlike his other daughters who, despite condescending to his ideas, instead looked on him with suspicion and without trust, for he had become so odious and bitter. Tara thought that if he agreed, her mother would be no problem.

It was the perfect moment for her request; perhaps, for once, her father would understand. When she explained the situation to him he just stared at her, confused, not knowing whether to get angry or how to react at all. Luckily for her she had never mentioned the word "warrior," instead speaking only of a "dance and exercises," for she knew that her father thought a woman should have nothing to do with war or any of its activities: such "honor" was destined only for men.

To Tara's surprise her father agreed. After all, he thought, it might do his daughter some good to learn this dance or whatever it was, for she had always been a good daughter, and seeing her so enthusiastic and happy at the idea, against all logic and tradition, he could not refuse. However, so his wife would be at peace with the idea, he named some conditions. On hearing them Tara's mother agreed, placing some conditions of her own. Both of them made Tara promise to ask the stranger certain questions before commencing her lesson the next afternoon.

Tara shone with happiness. She could not explain, but at last she felt as if she wanted to live again, and she could wait no longer to begin her lessons. The next morning she completed all of her chores earlier than usual and, as the appointed time approached, she prepared in a hurry, choosing comfortable clothes in which she could move easily and running to the place where they had agreed to have their first meeting.

She arrived early, and her future teacher was already there. It was clear that he had finished cleaning the flat area in front of the barn, freeing it from the occasional weed, stone, and fallen branch that might interrupt the process of a class.

She greeted him cordially and he answered in the same way.

"Welcome, Tara! I see you are ready for your first class, and I trust that your father has given you his approval . . . or no?"

She answered a little nervously. "Well yes . . . it's only that he and my mother have requested that I ask you some questions, to learn more of the nature of your teachings and of your intentions. Would you mind if I asked them?"

"And what if I do not wish to answer?"

"Perhaps they will be angry and not let me come again." She continued confidently, "But I would come anyway! It has been several years since I have been old enough. And besides, in a certain way I have already had my authorization and have done as you requested."

The man laughed, thinking that, in truth, the girl was insistent beyond anything he could have ever imagined. Immediately he replied, more seriously.

"All right, Tara, I will not place that inconvenience upon you. There is no reason that I should go against your parents; that has never been my intention. Ask me their questions."

She smiled.

"Well, my father, before settling down was a pilgrim much like yourself, and he understands a little of arts and teaching systems; at the same time, he and my mother have been faithful and true to the ways and beliefs of our ancestors. My mother, though a simple woman and devoted housewife, is a descendant of the ancient and renowned Eagle Clan. Because of this she is proud and apprehensive about her descendants. I mentioned that the name of your teaching is Boabom, and they said they had never heard such a name and could not imagine what it was all about, so they asked their questions."

"Go on, ask them, and be in peace with yourself and your parents."

"My father has four questions for you. First, he asked what the origin of your teaching was, then who your master had been and if you were one, what your lineage was, and, finally, why no one knows your Art."

The old wanderer answered immediately. "Your father is an intelligent and cautious man. It is no inconvenience to me to answer him; perhaps, however, he will find inconvenience at listening to my answers." He paused before calmly continuing.

"My answer is the following: tell him that the origin of my teaching is as old as these mountains, and the place from which it comes is beyond time and the eons, that from your perspective such a place is missing, leaving only the memory I carry, which is my Art. Tell him that this place, forgotten by time and the thoughts of men, has been called the Valley of the Mmulmmat, that some knew and named it as the Valley of the Warm Breeze or the Valley of the White Waters. Considering that such a place is not at the reach of anyone, I shall say that my teachings are orphaned in their origin, and considering that this Art has no nation, country, or village that your father can know or imagine, it can be said with certainty that it simply never belonged to any place, to any country or village, as the air, the fire, or the earth belong to no nation or human being, though so many waste their lives in such pretension.

"As for your second question, on who my master was and if I am one, listen carefully to what I will say. First, you shall know that the one who taught me was no master in the total sense that your father asks, and poorly could one who is not a master generate one, and therefore, neither am I one." The young woman stared at him in surprise, and he continued. "I must tell you that the one who taught me, as I too, would never allow that attribution of master, and would accept neither any reverence nor allow any kind of image to be adored, admired, or worshipped. Because this teaching, our Art, is a form that will allow you to find your own essence, meanly could those who cultivate it dedicate themselves to making images to be followed, admired, and they to be called masters by others. Your world is already plagued with saviors and masters; be considerate and do not add me or my predecessor to that long sad list.

"As for the name of the one who taught and opened the doors of Boabom to this old man, I cannot tell you, for that is a subject dealt with only between the one who teaches and the trusted apprentice, not with everyone. For now, as an answer, I can say that it was a woman, like yourself." Tara's mouth gaped in amazement, for she had never imagined that a woman could teach something such as this. The wanderer continued. "And besides, a name that you do not know will not tell you or your father anything new. Of that person you can know only part of the consequence of her pilgrimage, which is me, and now you. Her name shall pass into oblivion, just as mine shall pass . . . as will all those who are named. Inevitably shall it be forgotten, the voice by which they were titled, and they will be re-membered only by their real and daily actions and for the inevitable consequences that were born and shall be born out of the conse-quences of their actions.

"As for my lineage and my Art, you must know that we do not have such a thing, for neither my Art nor myself believe in any line-age. In such a way have passed those who, in their invisible way, have preceded me, and so shall pass all those who follow this Way, for you must understand that an apple tree produces such sweet fruits not because it was named apple tree or because it comes from others called the same, but for the invisible actions that make it, be-yond any named lineage that attempts to justify its quality. Besides, I could hardly transmit or explain to you and your father my lineage if I will not tell you the unknown name of the one who taught me.

But do not worry, for to the one who sees with trust, in a pure way, none of this is relevant. For the one who wants recognition, proof, to brag with trophies and awards with which they can prove their lack of falsity and excess of authenticity, this Art is not helpful. They must look for something that will enrich them on the outside as well as it impoverishes them on the inside. A great lineage! A great empty shell! Being so, if you become my student, you will barely know my name, and when you see me no more, you shall forget it so as not to forget me.

"Now you shall meditate on what I have said, and if you truly understand it, you will know the answer to your father's last question, why no one knows this teaching. If you have paid attention you will see that Boabom is a delicate Art, fine—so delicate and fine that, for this reason, you cannot see it. It belongs to the Clan of the Lonely, to those teachings whispered in someone's ear, and therefore its sounds are lost to those who are not in the right place or time to hear. You must understand that its name has gone unnoticed because this has always been its nature, its form, and its Way. If you have the opportunity to learn it now, this is something exceptional: simply take it, and if you are able, discover its secrets and its hidden name. If not, just leave me and continue with your life."

After a pause, the Wanderer continued.

"Meditate on all I have said, for there are things that are born, live, and exhaust each moment of their existence to be acknowledged and admired, and they are happy to have people gossiping about them; there are those who say they would do anything for others with the same simulated pretension, and there are those who think themselves safe in serving lords whom they will never meet, about whom they will hear only their names and their serious concern to never be forgotten by their servants. They all seek something that has no substance, give time for the external, but none have time for themselves; should they not begin with that? Thus, they win in appearance, win others or win their lords, but they lose themselves, and with that they lose the beautiful details that life gives to us without asking anything in return.

"If you follow this path, do so for yourself, and leave behind you any idea of satisfying others, or of winning their recognition or admiration."

Tara listened attentively, thinking that this man was truly wise, that he knew just what he was saying, and why he was saying it. All she wanted to do right then was to begin her classes as soon as possible, but she did not want to go against the wishes and curiosities of her mother, so she asked, timidly: "Truly, your answer belongs to a wise man, and even though my only desire is to be your student and begin with your teaching, I could not go home in peace without an answer to the four questions that my mother has asked."

"Go on, Tara," he calmly answered. "I have asked for this authorization from your parents in the belief that you would not so much as dare to ask them, or that if you did, your father would become so angry that I would never see you here again interrupting my practices, or that your mother would impose her doubts, and the fear that would fill you would be so great you would never come back to see me or to ask any teaching of me. Yet you have shown me that you truly want to learn, and that despite their doubts, your parents are essentially kind, and that they have given you a chance. That being so, I must aid you and give answers that you may take and transmit to them. I do hope that my answers will be useful and not disturbing, but I cannot contravene reality; just as you, your parents shall take them or leave them. Now, tell me what your mother has asked."

The young woman felt encouraged by what he said, though she sensed that, as he was warning her, perhaps her father and mother would not like his answers.

"My mother has four things she would like to know about: first, about your original language and your family; second, what of your gods and the writings on which they are based; third, how do you pray; and last, what are your plans or goals for the future."

He answered calmly, without any hint of annoyance or upset. "I can see that your mother too is a very intelligent person, and she certainly knows what to ask. Tell her this:

"About my original language and my family, you shall know, of the first, that it has been long since I have forgotten about it, that what I remember now is that I speak the language of movement, the one transmitted through the sounds made when my Art cuts the wind and when its dance expands in the three higher syllables: the inhalation, the containing, and the exhalation. That the words of this language are universal, for wherever I go, they can be spoken, understood, and learned easily; that its verses and sentences are dictated by vision, and it is always clean and lucid in its feeling and expression. Tell her that I speak the language that does not translate the words hatred or love, young or old, woman or man, caste or nation, flag or gods. Tell her that I speak the code of Boabom, which is intelligible only to those who understand the depths of its dance." After a short pause he added, opening his folded arms and looking at his limbs, "Besides, both you and she shall learn that this is my family, that each of its members travels always with me, and that my devotion to it is so great, so absolute, so delicate and inevitable that when she dies, I will die in the same moment.

"As for my gods, tell her that I do not possess gods, that I do not possess altars or relics. Yet if for her peace of mind, inevitably that a man of good should possess some kind of god, tell her that this shall be a silent goddess whose name I do not know." He gazed at the fields and then up to the skies as he continued. "About writings, simply look around you: here are the writings in which I am based. They are full of truths both hidden and obvious, possessing more pages than any of the others, pages that are never undone but always transform themselves to show you one revelation after another. If you are studious, watchful, and attentive, you will be able to decipher its sacred words; if you are careless, you will not perceive its form. If your mind is pure and lively, you will see it is filled with verses of happiness; if your mind is obtuse and negative, you will feel each of its dictates a cruel and unjust sentence. Yet in the end, in one way or another, with one vision or another, inevitably you will be ruled by its designs.

"Being so, my prayers seem strange to the religious, are ineffable to the mystics, incomprehensible to those who call themselves spiritual. But for your mother's comfort and for your own, I shall tell you that I pray daily and with absolute devotion, and that my prayers are thrown to the heights through my Art; that each time I deepen myself within it I enlighten the great altar with the most clean and tranquil fire, I burn incense of the finest perfume that could ever exist, while to it I dictate the most devoted and beautiful prayers. That these prayers give me flourishing health, a mind full of lucidity and joy, a flexible and strong will. Tell her that after these moments, everything shines within me and everything flourishes around me in an incredible happiness. What more than this can be asked of a real prayer?

"Last, your mother has wisely asked what are my goals. What is a man without goals? She shall say . . . 'Does not everything have a goal?' No doubt she believes that a man who has no goals is a man who cannot be trusted. She is correct,"—and he looked straight into Tara's eyes—"so tell her that for now, my goal is to able to make it through this winter while I await the opening of the passes, and meanwhile to teach to my student the Art that I carry, and then to continue with my pilgrimage . . . in peace."

Tara felt deeply touched by his answers, as if something that had always been there was coming to life within her. Then she thought, and worried, about what her parents might say; what made her more anxious, however, was knowing with certainty that she could begin the lessons.

The old man quickly told her that there would be no more lessons for that day; that he had granted her too much already, giving her answers that her parents demanded, and that now was the proper moment for her to leave and bring the answers to her parents. If all went well, he would await her the next day, to definitively begin with Boabom. She would still have to follow all of the rules he had mentioned in the beginning.

Tara felt disappointed, yet she understood the situation. She respectfully bid the old man good-bye and hurried back home.

When she returned, everything was the same. First she saw her mother, who asked her how the class had gone and what the strange teacher had said about the questions. Tara was about to begin her answer when at that very moment her father arrived, as usual a little bit drunk.

Tara began the explanation, transmitting what she had heard. From the beginning her mother did not like the answers very much, for she found them unclear, not concrete as she had wanted to hear. Her doubt began to turn into disgust and suspicion.

At the same time her father began laughing out loud. "Hahaha-hahahah! What a pilgrim," he said. "I like him, after all. He might be crazy or a wise man—isn't it the same?" Then he added, a little sad, "Well, am I just a sentimental old drunk or a stupid old man as my wife and daughters think?"

Her mother replied, "I do not like the idea of her being the student of this stranger, this unknown man. Besides, she should already be engaged, willing to marry and have children, and not learning strange things from a foreigner."

The father intervened immediately, not knowing if his answer was moved by reason or by the spontaneity of being drunk. "I like this Nnu-Suto a lot! Though I don't know him, I like his answers—hehehe—he very politely sent us to the hills! And we deserve it! Hahaha . . . you have my permission, Tara, and we won't speak of it anymore. Do as you wish, for you have your father's authority."

Her mother grumbled something before adding, "All right . . . it's all right. If your father says so, I accept it." And inside of her, she thought, *Well, if it's like he says, and a woman taught him, well then, he can't be such a bad man. . . .*

Chapter 4

THE THOUSAND WAYS OF BOABOM

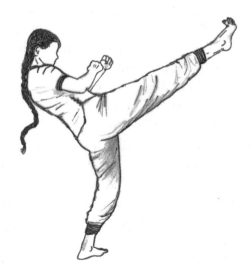

*You might forget your name
but you won't forget Boabom.*

—Nnuya, *"The Smith,"*
from The Legend of the Mmulmmat

TARA WOKE very early the next morning so that she could finish all of her work: in the house, in the family fields, and especially with the few animals they still had. Following the instructions of her strange teacher, she ate early and prepared comfortable clothes in which she could perform the movements without problems.

It was already afternoon when she came, a little early, for her first lesson. She ran up to the place where they were to have classes. Since it was cool and seemed that it might rain, the pilgrim was waiting inside the barn; she noticed him and entered, greeting him respectfully.

The man answered kindly, saying, "I can see you have had no inconvenience with your family, and that you are ready, even excited, about your first lesson."

Happy and relieved, Tara answered. "I am, honorable Nnu-Suto; I am prepared."

"Well," he said, smiling, "today this small barn will be appropriate for your learning."

"Will we be comfortable here?" she asked.

The wanderer answered in an understanding yet firm manner.

"First, know that my Art can be developed and learned in any place, that even though there are many who believe that external luxury and material abundance can improve the quality of a teaching, they are wrong. Luxury or material things you will always be able to find; if wisdom were so common as material things, it would be easy to discover, yet this is not so. Our Art can flourish in any place, large or small, comfortable or rough, with great resources or with great lack, yet always on the condition that wherever its seed may fall, it shall be the right soil, meaning that it shall be valued, and paid the attention and care that it requires. Therefore do not confuse values with luxury, do not see pure energy as similar to success, do not hope for internal achievements through titles and trophies. Pay attention to all that I explain, for even if you may think that what I shall teach are simple exercises and movements, you shall know that they are knitted together with these thoughts I have been transmitting to you."

He paused for a moment before continuing in a more kindly tone. "Today, you deserve this teaching, for somehow you have inquired after it, searched for it, and made a real effort to reach it. Your initial curiosity was simple. You brought a present without even knowing me or expecting anything of me, and you were brave, asserting what you feel while those around you doubted; this is why you deserve this teaching. Yours is the right soil, the proper field. The crops that we shall cultivate and harvest will depend on your determination, strength, and persistence over time."

Feeling happier and more enthusiastic with each word, she spoke. "I am anxious to begin! Do you think I should know more before I begin in order to better understand what you will teach me today?"

"Mmm . . . I see that you truly wish to understand this Art. All right. You have earned a detailed explanation of the principles of this teaching, and whenever you shall practice them, you shall know what thread you are weaving and thus what shape your fabric will acquire."

The wanderer took a single step and, with an elegant gesture, invited the young woman to sit. She made herself comfortable as the teacher, still standing, continued with his explanation.

"Listen carefully, for I shall reveal the earliest secrets of my teaching. I will tell you first that Boabom is a key word, summarizing many teachings, each of which, with your eyes, could be seen as different from the others. Its beginning rests in three fundamental Arts. Each of them possesses its own forms of movement, its own ways of execution and of how to value them, its own breathing techniques, its own short-term objectives and long-term goals, all of which work together. At the same time each of these Arts is developed as the construction of a building: each has its own base—which must be well structured and strongly built—and on this lie the main beams, and on them the other beams that will support the roof and walls. Finally, the details and adornments will be added to make it comfortable."

As he explained all of this, the mysterious man gestured gracefully with his hands and cast his face into various expressions; it was these that most caught the attention of the student.

"These three fundamental Arts," he continued, "have their own warmup and stretching systems, as well as their own technical development, and for this reason it is said that we should not speak of three Arts but of six. Yet do not be confused by such numbering because I shall explain what I mean by this, for it will be good for you to understand that this teaching involves many branches, which are clearly subdivided, and clearly you should know on which of these branches you are beginning to tread this winter. Simply stated, all of these teachings constitute Boabom, and it is through this name that I shall explain their development.

"So Boabom, as I was saying, has three fundamental branches. Allow me to enumerate them for you.

"First, **Gentle Boabom,** which we refer to technically as **Seamm-Jasani,** is the first of its branches. But as I was just saying, each system has a double form of development; thus Seamm-Jasani consists of two clearly distinct stages.

"The first of these is the **Jass-U of Seamm-Jasani,** which we also call the Art of Osseous Awakening, since this stage teaches simple and gentle stretches, exercises, breathing techniques, and movements of relaxation, all of which would seem to be the kind of movements one should do just after waking from sleep. As you know, when we awake in the morning our movements are slowed and a little clumsy; this is the reason for my example. Our energy needs first to know the way . . . to wake up! It is after this stage that we learn the:

"**Seamm-Jasani** itself, called also the Art of Eternal Youth. It consists of gentle, soft techniques and coordinations, as well as basic meditation, which require a lot of patience. The development of this form allows the student to strengthen the weaknesses inherent in the whole body, increasing its longevity while learning or forming the channels in which the other branches will run, so that these are more easily understood."

After a short pause for the student to digest what he had said, he continued.

"As you can see, this first form is a complete teaching within itself. Owing to the nature of how it generates heat and because it ignites slowly yet at the same time burns for a long time in its generation, we can compare it to the heat of charcoal.

"On a parallel level we have a second form, which we can consider as a sister, or a reflection, of the previous, but from a distant angle.

"This is the second Art, or **Osseous Boabom.** Because of its central importance, its difficulty, and that it is the most fundamental foundation of all these teachings involving movement, we name it directly **Boabom.** It too has two fundamental forms that every student must understand.

"**Jass-U of Boabom,** to which we attach the name the Art of Osseous Awakening, as it shall form and prepare the structure of the body for the solid movements of Boabom. As the Gentle way develops its own awakening, this current stage works in the same way, though from another perspective we assume that the body has already the condition for a relatively rigorous demand. This branch has its own techniques of breathing, its own warming and stretching systems, which act both quickly and with strength, traveling from the head to the toes, preparing the student's physical and vital structure for the demands that the second, or technical, part demands. Think now that you will do the movements of this technical cycle at a speed so sparkling and precise that, if done wrong, they could easily turn against you. Thus this stage of awakening is necessary, so the heavier meal will not be poorly digested. As we see and live this in practice you will better understand what I am explaining now. It is then from this stage that we move immediately to the next:

"**Osseous Boabom,** which we also call, symbolically, the Art of the Thousand Ways, or more simply the Osseous Art. To superficial eyes this would seem a singular Art of defense, and it is this that you have seen me doing in those times when you were secretly watching me. Through this branch is developed the most essential vitality, the depth of spontaneous movement, and its development is as solid and demanding as it is incommensurable. Its movements, as you will see, are characterized by sagacity, skill, self-control: its speed in sparks like lightning falling from a clear sky, without warning, or like those things you have seen come from your clothes when you are in the mountains and the weather is extremely dry.

"It is characterized also by its study and development of reflection, and also by its precision: the mechanics, spontaneity, and invisibility in the development of the technique. Each movement can have a double or triple meaning. You will see too that it finds its main energy source in breathing, and that it can be used as a way to control concentration, tiredness within your own mind, and the projection of the most solid internal energies that act in conjunction with each movement. This Art carries a direct relation to the confidence that each being can develop, its hidden strength, for though it is like a dance projected as a precise and extraordinary form of defense, at the same time it studies the awakening of the inner forces, or vortices, of the magnetic field. The movements develop intertwined, forming a chain, an infinite continuity of thousands of techniques: circular, oblique, straight, retractile, spiral-shaped, and in the higher circle of the thirty-three tips.

"I am certain that much of what I am explaining you will not understand, but anyway I take the time to tell you all of this, for each word will be recorded in your mind, and as you advance in this Art, you will discover for yourself what I meant with all of these expressions. For those who do not walk the path, these words will remain simply the 'crazy' utterances of another wanderer, and nothing more. That is how it shall be, for only the one who perseveres deserves to understand the true meaning and symbolism of these words.

"Know also that, because of the way that this system produces heat, and of the explosion of energy it produces in the student, we link it to a great bonfire of dry wood, which burns fast and with great intensity.

"Now, and only as a passing interest, I will speak to you of the third branch, to which I have referred earlier in my conversation. It is generally classified as one of the higher branches, as its learning presupposes that the student have a certain antiquity within Osseous Boabom. It is called:

"**Boabom of Elements,** whose more direct name is Yaanbao. This form is born from the previous ones, yet it too had its own development and life. Within it is studied movement extended by different elements, formed as sticks of varying sizes: medium, long, short, as well as other shapes. It too is divided into two main stages:

"**Jass-U of Yaanbao,** which could be called the Art of Osseous Awakening for Elements. Through this come the movements necessary for the student to become familiar with the various elements that he or she shall learn to handle. These elements complement the application of exercises and breathing techniques. From this one is born:

"**Yaanbao** itself. This system seeks to perfect the strength and confidence of the student. One path has been the gentle one, the other learning and putting into practice speed and reaction; this branch perfects the movement with speed applied to elements that will work in harmony with the prepared student yet will act coldly against the amateur, who is neither dedicated nor firm enough. The Yaanbao is the study of inertia and the force of the elements. Its development is acquired in stages, each of which works with different sizes and shapes of elements.

"This challenging Art not only generates heat and an explosion of energy but at the same time demands the maximum attention of the student, and as it empties it renews from within. For this reason we can see it as a caged bonfire, or the continuous and dangerous burning produced by the wood located in a great siphon."

After a pause, the teacher continued with his explanation while the student gave her full attention.

"Finally, these first two main branches work and are developed independently, even though, as I have said before, with the third they form one grand fabric. And you shall learn that there are many other branches or forms that I have not named, for which you are not yet prepared. But the proper occasion will come. If this comes to be so, you will see why I have spoken of one Art with many branches.

"This teaching, what I shall give and you shall receive, this method, this Way in which I shall guide you, this forms our own school between you, this old man, and what he carries. This bond, this nexus we call Mmulargan. Be happy, for there is a current of learning, and if there is the movement of transmission, then there is energy . . . thus there is a life being generated . . . to evolve!"

As he finished speaking, Nnu-Suto made an elegant gesture, calling his student to stand. She did this enthusiastically, excited to begin the practical stage. He spoke a few words as a final explanation.

"All right, Tara, you have been attentive and I hope I did not bore you too much with my explanation, but it is necessary that you know the basics, the fundamental development of what you are to learn and of what you have earned for yourself. Finally, however, I shall clarify for you that, of these three branches I should begin with the first of them, the gentle stages, yet I sense that this winter will be a short one, and I can feel that your character is strong and full of vitality, as is your body. Thus I shall take the risk of directly initiating you into Boabom, the Osseous Art. I am also aware that your essence is combative and curious, so I take the risk of teaching you this stage, but remember your promise not to use it."

She nodded silently.

"Remember that Boabom will quickly develop a great energy within you. This energy, in its physical stage, will be quickly reflected in movements that, as I have said before, can be seen as a dance yet which possess a thousand faces that can easily transform into a silent defense, more real and effective than you can imagine."

Tara continued in her silent waiting, listening as her desire to begin continued to grow. This strange man had truly managed to feed her curiosity each and every moment, and this continued as he completed his explanation.

"Well . . . now you must follow me and imitate my movements: in the beginning we will see the first part of Osseous Boabom, the Jass-U or preparatory stage, which consists of simple exercises. Do not take them lightly, though; instead be careful and precise in your practice. Later, once we have warmed our bodies, we will begin the second stage, the Technical Boabom. Today you will see the base of both of these. After the class be sure to keep yourself well warmed and to clean yourself in the heat of your house, with warm water heated over the fire, making sure not to let yourself get cold. Though it is cold outside this afternoon, we will be generating a great heat, capable even of melting snow and hard ice! Yet even when we become capable of that within our Art, we must never abuse this or try to prove anything, for such things are not necessary. Now, relax and follow me. If I make a sound that reminds you of a kind of counting, it is to help you to follow the rhythms appropriate to each movement; just follow that rhythm. Those sounds I will make are key words, or mantras, as you might call them. They exist to center the mind and develop your energy to the maximum."

With shining eyes, Tara was as happy as she was curious. Somehow that man was revealing before her an unknown world, beyond the paths blocked by the snows, beyond the routine of daily work. In that moment she felt that she was in the Valley of the Warm Breeze that he had named as the origin of his Arts.

Nnu-Suto then made a curious gesture in the air with his hands united, and the class began immediately. First, as he had told her he would, he showed her short movements that would serve to quickly awaken and heat her muscles and joints. As quickly as he had begun these, he stopped to explain the breathing technique. This Guide was very precise in his explanations, and he showed her how to do each movement, and how not to. In that way she understood perfectly the correct application and development of each movement. The exercises were simple: first he did them slowly, so she could easily understand, then he increased the speed, demanding the maximum of her, yet they never lost the rhythm of the breathing. She was surprised, for she had never thought she could sweat so much or feel so much heat in her body while everything around her seemed cold and damp. It seemed to her as if the sun was shining directly on her head, on one of those days where the heat was caged within the mountains.

And she saw, too, the grace with which the old teacher moved, and he did not seem so old anymore.

Soon they were finished with the first part, and they moved directly into the second stage. Now Nnu-Suto's explanations had even more detail: first he showed her a basic position in the shape of an arch, which he explained was the most simple and that this was why it was called Universal Position. He explained too that this position would give her stability and make her feel solid, yet he said that in the future they would forget this position, for there were many others she had to learn and they would end up replacing this. Then he showed her the basic hand positions, and finally the first hand projection, which he called The Force of the Spiral. The Guide explained to her that this was only the beginning, that it was nothing compared to what was yet to come. He also showed her how this final movement projected all of the energy through the arm in a fearsome spiral, ending in the eruption of what he called the twin volcanoes, or the two primary knuckles: the bases of the index and middle finger.

After they had spent some time in studying and applying the first movements of Boabom, the student was covered in sweat: her face was red and her expression was one of complete happiness. Somehow, already she began to better understand this strange pilgrim.

Finally, Nnu-Suto finished the lesson, uniting his hands again, in a way to seal the teachings of that day. He briefly explained some details to her, then left his student free to go. Yet she stood, without a word; she felt full of energy, despite the rigor of the lesson.

"Have you any doubts or questions?" he asked.

"Yes! I would like to know how I should refer to you, since you are not . . . you are not a master."

"Good question," answered the Teacher. "If you like, you can call me directly Nnu-Suto. Or you can also call me Guide, for as such I shall show and conduct you in Boabom; later you will come to your own conclusions. I will simply be a bridge."

She smiled, again liking his explanation. "I am very thankful, Guide Nnu-Suto, for your teaching. I hope to be a good student."

"Welcome, Tara! What will be will be! Now go home and rest, for you are free to go! Remember that you must take care of yourself, especially from the cold; I will wait for you here, no matter what happens, the day after tomorrow. If your muscles feel a little sore or tired, do not worry—just remember the hot water. Now go, go!"

She said nothing; by instinct she made a quick respectful gesture before running home, full of joy.

Chapter 5

OSSEOUS

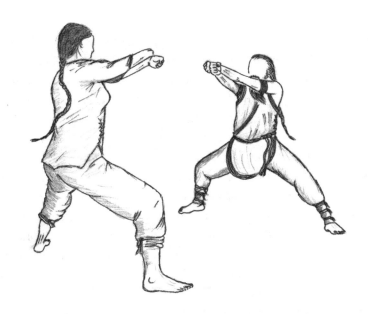

Patience . . . Everything has its time;
for now knit, just knit; be an Artisan of the Mind.

—*Alsam, from* Bamso, the Art of Dreams

WINTER BEGAN to slowly cast its white and magical veil over the mountains. With every lesson, Tara went deeper into the movement, the technique, and every last detail of the mysterious Osseous Art that the lonely wanderer continued to transmit to her.

Meanwhile, at home everything moved along at its normal pace. Her parents were a little surprised, however, at the constantly increasing optimism they began to see in her. Without even noticing it herself, the previously introverted and taciturn young woman was left in the past. Her sisters only watched, chattering amongst themselves.

On the other hand, the small town was giving renewed meaning to the phrase "small town, big hell." Many of the neighbors began spreading rumors that were, in general, not so well intentioned; for them, the continued presence of the pilgrim was strange and uncomfortable. Some wondered if he was a deserter from a far-off war, while others said that he must have been a bandit lost in the loneliness of the mountains. Still others even ventured that he might be a wizard who practiced strange arts and cast curses and that, because of this danger, his presence was in no way good for the already suffering village. Although, in fact, this last kind of rumor made the old man feared and respected as well, for who would dare to speak badly of a wizard? He might become angry and unleash a hailstorm over the next year's crops or cause the cattle to wander and die, lost and frozen.

Yet those who housed him remained pleased with his presence; to them he seemed a kind old man, and he had paid the agreed rent on time. What they liked best about him, though, was that he paid with small gold nuggets and fine gems that actually exceeded the value of what he was renting.

Tara only shrugged her shoulders at such rumors as the villagers spread: she was so engrossed in what she was learning that she barely had time to listen to the old ladies' chatterings. She had lived her whole life in that village and knew perfectly that mentality; she was accustomed to such gossiping about one neighbor, and the next week about another. Besides, the recent war and the year's poor harvest and shortages had made all of them more susceptible.

As the winter began, she was moving deeper into this Boabom Art; without intention, she often discovered herself practicing the different techniques while feeding the livestock or doing her daily activities. On more than one occasion her father watched her from a distance: he knew this was the strange dance the foreigner was teaching her. Deep within himself he also knew that the teaching was more profound than it seemed, and he knew that this Art was unique, the likes of which he had never seen before, and that it doubtless contained shades of some rare forms of defense, dance, and relaxation. In silence he felt proud of his daughter's stubbornness and, also in silence, he tried to imitate what she did, making sure that she did not notice. Through all of this, he wisely kept his own counsel, saving his thoughts for himself; for he wanted neither to feed the fire of the town's gossip nor to have it said that Tara was becoming some sort of mystical warrior.

Days, then months passed. One afternoon Tara went punctually, as she always did, to her class in the barn. The place had slowly become accustomed to its new use. Tara and her teacher had repaired the decrepit roof and walls. They had also leveled the ground that served as its floor, and now it was easy for them to practice the movements in a more free and open way.

That afternoon Nnu-Suto was, as usual, smiling and in a good mood. They greeted each other respectfully and, before beginning the lesson, he asked her: "How have you felt, advancing within the Art? Has it been worthwhile?"

"Of course!" she answered, enthusiastic. "Just as you said, as the classes have gone on, I have felt better, and even though I sweat a lot and the lessons can be demanding, once we finish the class I feel excellent and return home full of energy for my work. From your advice I have realized that this energy is very personal: I would love for this whole village to feel it, but I am aware that this cannot be. I only try to enliven everyone as best I can. But anyway . . . what is really important is that I can continue learning!"

"Has anything else called your attention?"

"There is something else . . . really that always surprises me, and it is that I am always learning something new; I can tell that you truly dislike routine. The other day I heard one of the young men who went to war with my brothers; he is always boasting, swaggering around, and he was saying that when he was off on the battlefield he met a true master of martial arts, who had proven that the only way to learn was by repeating the same punch hundreds of times, just as he could harden himself by placing his hands in hot sand, breaking bricks, stones, or large branches against his stomach and head, or bathing for hours under the frigid waterfalls of the fresh thaw. When I heard this, I thought of how you had never said any such thing and that always, in every class, you teach me something new, so your Art quickly changes, and more than just a group of techniques it seems to grow, and evolve . . . will it always be like this?"

Nnu-Suto smiled as he quietly answered Tara. "Your perspective about this teaching is opening slowly, Tara, and now you are prepared for me to explain it in more detail. What I shall now tell you will clear your doubts, but to confirm it . . . you must continue your learning and live these things for yourself, as only you can validate how much truth there is in my words or likewise in the words of anyone else. Always remember that there is nothing more wise or correct than your own experience." The Guide took a breath before continuing. "You must be clear that, as you have lived it, two roads, or main threads, constitute Boabom: as I have told you before, one is the Jass-U of Boabom, while the other is Boabom itself. Now let me explain in detail the development of each one, so you will understand this clearly and therefore understand how this Art is, its birth, life, and plenitude, and how, beginning from this, Boabom is reflected in the union of body and mind, not against it.

"First, we will analyze the **Jass-U,** or the **Art of Osseous Awakening.** You will have appreciated that it begins and develops quickly, and that at the same time it has its own divisions, of which you have seen three main threads.

"The first thread is formed by the **Standing Movements** (Cycle 1), the second by the **Movements on the Floor** (Cycle 2), and the third by the **Final and Closing Movements** of this stage (Cycle 3).

"Now you will be able to understand the specifics of my explanation, as you have experienced these three stages in your classes. Thus, the **First Cycle** encompasses the main exercises to awaken your limbs and torso. First and most simple was to learn how to stand in a relaxed way, the torso straight but without exaggeration. We generated a Base Position and, starting from this initial balance, we could easily develop the rest of the exercises. The movements then began with the low zone, the legs, vigorously infusing them with heat and energy. We have seen too a basic breathing technique, which we have called the Breathing Technique of Inner Power. We have called it this because, on the one hand, this technique helps us to control our tiredness, to better feed or provision us with energy, while on the other hand it makes all of the weak and vulnerable points strong, even though this sounds incredible. You shall know that this strengthening must not be seen only as a shield or defense but also as a way to revitalize the internal organs, stimulating and exercising them. Last, this First Cycle follows another sequence, providing the necessary heat and energy to the different regions of the body: legs, knees, feet, arms, elbows, hands, and wrists, and to the trunk in general. Immediately from this, we cultivate the second cycle of the Osseous Jass-U.

"The **Second Cycle** concerns movements executed on the floor. We continue here in a new sequence of exercises done seated or lying down, which focus generally on the abdomen and also on basic forms of stretching. As you know already, each movement within this stage, just as in the previous one, is quick, constant, and executed with energy, for this is how everything is within Boabom: a great bonfire! Also, in this stage we learn the basic hand positions that we eventually use in Osseous Boabom. From this point we move to the final part, and from there to the closing, which together form one cycle.

"The **Third Cycle,** in which we stand again, concerns itself with the final stages of stretching. This cycle reactivates the legs, in order to prepare us to learn the more technical Osseous Art. We finish this cycle by twice repeating the Breathing Technique of Inner

Power, with which our body and mind will be ready to continue learning.

"You will have noticed that *I did not* teach all of this system to you in your first class, but that I showed only a few of its elements, although I did begin with the Breathing Technique of Inner Power, for all of our movements are based upon it. With each class we added new movements from all three cycles until, by the end of the first month, we had completed this pattern of the three cycles of the Osseous Jass-U.

"You probably have noticed that, parallel to this, in each class we have advanced in Boabom itself, adding one movement after another; in this way we have formed a chain or, better said, a fabric of movements.

"Now I will explain the second part in detail, so you can know how this teaching generates itself, continuous with the evolution of the body, not in opposition to it.

"**Boabom,** or the **Osseous Art,** possesses its own warp and weft, its own threads and unions of those threads. We have always referred to this Art by the term Osseous, for this, as you already know, forms the essential structure of its movement, or its medulla. From this point of view we can also compare it to a spine, for it is solid yet flexible, and though it may seem hard and defined, it is yet able to yield and adjust, having the qualities of endurance and strength of arches and natural curves. Finally, and just as any organism, it is alive and generates itself.

"In these months you have been developing the first stage of Boabom, which can be categorized in its own stages, too, though in the end it will constitute only one Great Movement. Allow me to explain and enumerate, step by step, these stages, for in the right moment, each detail I will tell you shall become useful to you.

"Stage I. Initial Positions: If you have been attentive, you may have realized that each movement has a base, or a form from which to begin. We have applied these from the very first classes, and with time you will see that they are of an infinite variety, even though we begin with the most simple. Of these initial positions you have come to know one, the Position of Rest and Discipline, which we have also called Osseous Field. It centers your energy, your magnetic field, and prepares your mind to focus completely on its learning. You have also learned Universal Position, or the arch, upon which we have built the next stage.

"Stage II. Initial Hand Techniques: Within these we have learned, day by day, forms by which we project the hands; we have begun with the fist and its Twin Volcanoes. Recall that we have so called these points, actually your two main knuckles, for they are both connected directly to the osseous structure of the hand and forearm, which means that they have a great, solid base, like a pair of mountains. We call them Volcanoes for, as such, they can transmit a very hot energy when used correctly in projection, even more when used in the spiral of energy you have learned bit by bit. Keep this technique secret, for only the dedicated and studious will understand it; in the hands of an amateur it will turn against him. Also within this stage we have begun to use the projections with an open hand; however, you must be aware that we are only beginning and that what I have shown you thus far is nearly nothing.

"Stage III. Initial Techniques of Stepping and Their Application: Always, in every class, as you have understood the fundamentals of the previous movements, we have included the first steps you have taken within Boabom. This we have simply called the Path, which is a relatively simple position but essential in order to understand what shall come next. Over the course of its development we have learned and will continue to learn how to apply the different techniques, so as to patiently give life to each and every one of them.

"**Stage IV. Initial Foot Techniques:** Within this fourth stage, we have added movements of the feet and the legs, learning how to use them in a precise way, with fluidity, elegance, and yet finally with a speed that imitates lightning or the sharp movement of a powerful whip. With time, you will see that the movements of this kind are countless.

"**Stage V. Basic Study of the Forms of Reaction and Opposing Projection:** Now, as months have passed and you have begun to possess a solid base, feeling confidence with all of the previous stages, we can begin to delve into this stage. Here we put into practice the fundamental principle that 'every action brings a reaction.' Here we begin to apply the previous stages in a practical way, simulating a form of imaginary defense, which means, practically, the ways in which we can react, using the base of what we have learned so far, when faced with someone who projects and tries to strike you. But remember one thing: I am not a warrior, and poorly could I make one of you, for as I have said before, to make war you must first be at war within yourself, and the objective of my Art is totally the opposite. Therefore, learn these coordinations as a focused reaction and appreciate them simply as an exercise for your mind, for that is what they are. Isolate your mind through them, lay your instinctive fear aside, abandon your reasoning, and the spontaneous reaction will be born within you, for that is what we seek. Here the reflection is primarily stimulated by the sight, in order to reverse the action which is about to come. As you overcome yourself in this stage, your mind will be more fluid, simple, and confident.

"**Stage VI. Basic Study of the Forms of Reaction When**

Being Taken: Parallel to the previous stage, we will then learn bit by bit this other form of reaction; the difference between them is that these are used when we feel ourselves being taken and held, or grabbed, whatever the zone of the grab might be. Here the reaction is stimulated by tactile sensation, before we reverse the action, neutralizing and returning the energy needed for this effect. Meditate on this, too, for its proper practice will help you discover the instinctive self.

"**Final or Ending Stage:** In each class we complete a meditative closing, mentally reviewing our achievements and learning for that day. By this we acquire the learning totally, transforming it to be one with us, forcing it to give up its deepest secrets."

Tara listened attentively to these detailed descriptions as Nnu-Suto continued with his usual fluidity of speech and expression.

"By now you should know that everything I have taught you, and all that I am yet to teach, forms a fabric that grows, bit by bit, and does not stop. We will always learn something new: Boabom does not end in one life, for it is an Art for many lives! Each movement leads to a new one endlessly, thus by nature it is in motion. Now I can say one thing more directly to you, trusting that you have understood the true meaning of my words and teachings. It is this: that you have done well by making no comment whatsoever to the arrogant boy of whom you have spoken. It is normal for an arrogant person to follow another and imitate him, for magnets attract iron and not wood. This neighbor of yours who thinks, from what he has heard, that a body can be developed by the eternal repetition of one determined movement, has made a terrible and common mistake. The mind, as well as its physical manifestation the body, is infinite, and therefore the movements it can learn and develop are the same, just as in Boabom, where a new movement supports, develops, and perfects the older one. The only limit is your own patience, constancy, and search.

"Also, his comments about destroying objects in order to show strength, or challenging the elements of nature to show his superiority, or subjugation of himself—these are sadly mistaken. Our body is our most valuable tool, and we must care for it as best we can, giving it abundant positive energy. Its essence is soft and noble; why force it to face something hard that does us no harm? Why challenge the elements of nature if before them we are so small? Why is it better to not use our wisdom and intelligence to unite these elements that can help us in a generous way? Every unnecessary confrontation is motivated only by fear and ignorance of oneself, for nothing martial can be in any way related to an art, for this latter concept is one of creation, not of useless destruction or dispute."

After a short pause, the pilgrim glanced to his side, looking between the cracks in the barn at the moon, which on that day lay in sharp contrast to the blue afternoon sky above the mountains. He sighed and then spoke again. "Already in your past and perhaps in the future of those whom you do not yet know, there have been other wars, in a dimension far beyond your memories and time. Out of that ancient confrontation were born many of the mistakes you see around you. For example, from it comes the belief—how absurd—of vanquishing your body simply because of a so-called being, the spirit . . . but be patient, for someday you will understand." Nnu-Suto turned and spoke one last thing. "Well, it is already time for the practical, enough with too much theory. Let us move to our class! We must continue with our teachings, for you still have much to learn."

Tara smiled and prepared for her new lesson as, within herself, she tried to hold on to everything that she had learned.

The energy of the class itself was huge, and she understood, step-by-step, what they were doing, perfectly complementing Nnu-Suto's detailed descriptions. With intent, they reviewed the first Forms of Reaction and added new movements and techniques.

After about an hour the class was finished. At its end they meditated for a moment in tranquility and then respectfully said goodbye. Tara was drenched with sweat, and as usual her cheeks glowed an intense red. Before parting, she asked one thing.

"I have a concern, noble Nnu-Suto. If your Art does not end and grows ever greater and greater, and you are leaving as soon as winter ends, how will I continue learning?"

He smiled at her and said only, "Leave now, for it is late already . . . and you must prepare for tomorrow."

Chapter 6

FROM MOVEMENT TO INNER POWER

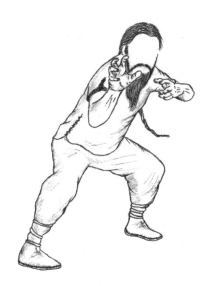

The energy and inner power need only a sparkle,
not a bonfire.

—*Jal, "The Black Amlom,"*
from The Legend of the Mmulmmat II

WINTER HAD ALREADY reached its peak, and as time passed, the teachings of Nnu-Suto flourished in his student with grace and virtue. She was very punctual in attending her classes, and on certain afternoons she made sure her teacher was well provisioned or took care that he was not cold, supplying him with the necessary comforts. She did her best to supply these things without upsetting her family, for the season was not very abundant. The fields, however, are always generous.

After some time the cold began to diminish, and slowly the temperature became more bearable. That winter Tara had noticed a significant change in her health: she caught no colds and did not become sick at any time through the whole season, and she no longer felt cold in her body, which was quite unusual. Also, she began to feel more confident, strong, and vigorous; somehow she was starting to live the effects of the Art. Something else, too, had called her attention, for her dreams had, bit by bit, evolved from total obscurity to a magical lucidity.

Despite this new positive experience, a thought troubled her more and more as the new season grew. The passes were beginning to clear, and she feared that soon the strange pilgrim would continue his journey. She did not wish even to mention this to him, for fear of reminding and thus encouraging him to take the initiative and continue his journey.

The village, as always, continued in its own rhythm. Her father still, from time to time, drowned the memory of his sons' deaths. Lately, though, and slowly, he had been drinking less. Yet one afternoon something strange occurred. The village was going on in its traditional routine: some of the women were working to move some animals, and a group of men had gathered in one of the houses to speak and while away the afternoon. From afar, the beats of horses' hooves could be heard, and as the sound came closer, the women outside stopped what they were doing, sensing that those approaching so rapidly were not of the village.

Almost immediately, four ferocious-looking men on horses appeared at the main entrance to the village, galloping and screaming senselessly. The women were frightened and froze where they were. No one knew who these men might be: victorious soldiers, renegades, or simply drunken bandits. Whichever they were, the villagers all stood, watching and waiting to see what would happen. Two of these unexpected visitors dismounted, swaggered close to a group of women gathered near the cattle, and began to harass them. No one did anything to defend the women: the men nearby neither moved nor seemed to have any intention to do so. Perhaps they feared that these intruders were really soldiers and that, if they said or did anything, there would be worse consequences. Perhaps they were simply afraid. Either way, while two of the intruders remained on their horses, the two dismounted men continued to torment the women, who were trying in vain to escape from a situation that was growing more frightening by the minute.

At this moment Tara and her father, who were walking down the nearby road, immediately noticed the trouble. He made a gesture to his daughter to stay behind as he walked forward with courage. He was a man of many battles and did not mind participating in yet another.

He walked quickly to one of the men and hit him with all his strength in the face. The man fell immediately, stunned. The second man, however, reacted roguishly, attacking Tara's father with a stick. He hit him in the head, and Tara's father fell to the ground, wounded. The attacker cackled at his quick success while his partner pulled himself up off the ground, and the two of them prepared to finish off the old man. Tara, however, could no longer remain uninvolved, and came alone to defend her fallen father. Seeing her come closer, the man with the stick tried to take her by the shoulders, from the front, but the girl quickly recalled what she had learned, taking a solid position while simultaneously projecting her crossed fists into her attacker's face. Then, in almost the same instant, she spread his arms, opening them as one opens two windows. After this, and with certainty, she used a quick leg projection, The High Whip Foot, which she joined with a strong breathing sound. She hit the man full in the face, and he was immediately thrown back, his stick and two of his teeth landing several feet away.

While this was happening, one of the mounted men had gotten down and, without Tara noticing, had snuck up behind her. He held her tightly while the second attacker came closer to her: his intentions were far from good. For a moment the girl felt defenseless, for it seemed impossible to free herself and no man from the village seemed to have any desire to rescue her. The man holding her began to laugh loudly. She inhaled and exhaled, trying to calm herself, and without thinking she reacted automatically, all of a sudden, and applied another Form of Reaction that she had learned: The Fish That Escapes. She lowered herself by gently bending her knees and, inhaling strongly, used a forward projection, The Force of the Double Spiral, which immediately released her from the bear hug and produced, at the same time, a noticeable effect on the facing attacker. Yet when she did this, she brought the movement back with a strong exhale, thrusting her elbows into the stomach of the one who had held her. Both men fell, suffocated by the strikes, and it seemed that all would end there. This, however, was not so.

The man with the stick, the first to have fallen, stood up again, still a little dazed but willing to continue the match. The fourth man, too, still on his horse, thought only of trampling Tara. But when he galloped toward her, something extraordinary happened.

Nnu-Suto appeared in the middle of the scene. He stood in front of Tara and simply stared into the eyes of the galloping man, who felt such great fear that he stopped his horse a few feet from the young woman and the Wanderer. The man with the stick, too, froze at the presence of the old pilgrim: cold shivers ran down his spine and he knew immediately that it was time to leave that village in peace. Tara was alert, but she was surprised by the attackers' sudden expression of fear. The man with the stick threw it down and began helping the two men on the ground to get up and onto their horses as quickly as possible. The four then left immediately, without looking back.

Everyone was astonished at the whole situation, at the courage of Tara and the magical way in which Nnu-Suto imposed his presence. No one said a word. After a moment some came silently and helped Tara's father, who had sustained quite a wound to his head.

A few days later Tara met with her teacher again in the barn. After their greetings, he inquired about her father's condition. She said that he was recovering, that he had been badly injured but that he was expected to recover soon. Nnu-Suto gave her some wild herbs that would help the old man recover, then said: "Give my best energies to your father, and say to him that I understand from where the courage of his daughter comes."

She lowered her head. "Are you not mad at me?" she asked, distressed. "I have used what you taught me, and I had promised not to."

"It is all right, Tara." Nnu-Suto spoke kindly. "I know that it was strictly necessary, that your father's physical well-being was endangered; that has justified your actions, just as your own defense would, especially if you have tried all the other possible options first."

The young woman, in brighter spirits now, replied. "I have a question. What did you do there to intervene and, without any movement, to make those fools leave so quickly."

"Eeeiii!" The pilgrim smiled as he answered, making a singular gesture. "A good Boabom Guide always keeps something for himself . . . hehehehe!"

So she was left with her terrible curiosity but did not dare insist, for she knew that he would continue joking and avoid the answer. Instead she changed the subject.

"Excuse me, noble Nnu-Suto, but I have remembered something."

She produced a basket that she had brought with her and quickly unwrapped something—inside was a big piece of freshly made cheese: she knew how Nnu-Suto loved it. The old man laughed again.

"Very good, Tara, very good. It seems that you already know my weak spots! Hehehe . . . I think that, after all, I will explain part of what I keep to myself, which will provide a cure for your curiosity. Come, sit down, and pay attention to what I am about to tell you."

The young woman sat quietly smiling, for she was about to learn something new about her mysterious teacher and his Art.

"Land, work, sowing, patience, and fruits!" said Nnu-Suto, as his student sat, attentive. "That is the law you have known since you were little, the way that these lands have taught you. You shall find that Boabom is the precious fruit that is achieved in this same way that your family gets its food each year. The chosen land, to which we have dedicated the necessary time and energy, which you have cultivated, planted your patience in, delivers its harvest in all shapes. In the same way our Art requires the same diligence and effort to reap its fruits, which with time become sweeter and more delicious.

"As for that, know that what you have learned so far covers only the first step of eight stages, each with its own fruits. After these eight fruits is born a higher stage, with newer achievements, and so on, to end in a state where the fruits and the labor to obtain them bear no difference from each other.

"I know that what I am explaining can be confusing; however, if you meditate on it and persist in Boabom, you will find the right time and proper solution for these examples. You shall also learn that since the students of this Art are a fruitful field and the teaching a well-selected seed, the harvest, the results, can go beyond common reason.

"Thus far you have been able to see Boabom as a form of defense, and even though this is only one of its faces, it is through this defense that I shall explain how the Art moves from mechanical to invisible . . . from movement to Inner power, which has so called your attention.

"Heed my words, for in Boabom there are three forms, or skeins of thread that form a triple braid, woven through all of its stages of teaching. These three forms are: the mechanical defense, or movement; the spontaneous defense; and the invisible defense, or Inner power. That day on which you saw the need to use what you have learned, the mechanical and spontaneous stages prevailed in you . . . and in me, the invisible stage prevailed. I am aware that this might surprise you, but if you are attentive and have a great dedication to this teaching, you will understand.

"Now, bring all of your senses to my explanation.

"The Exterior Movement, or Mechanical Defense, is manifested through the whole Art, indicating to us that its development is through techniques, steps, and projections in this state and physical dimension. You have learned from the first steps how to move your body, imitating me; you have learned to train it, strengthen it, coordinate it, make it have a certain harmony every time you apply each of its techniques. But the question is this: What part of you moves when you imitate each of the movements that I transmit? Is it your arm? Is it your breathing? Is it your muscles? The nerve that transmitted the instruction? Or the brain that dictated that instruction, stimulated by the senses? Through this simple riddle we can see that through one movement or technique of projection we have achieved the mind, and the organ through which it is manifested: the brain and its nervous extension. Every time we work with movements that are outside our routine, every time we need to coordinate them and apply them harmoniously, in unison with specific forms of breathing . . . you will be able to confirm with certainty that you have imitated a technique and, therefore, have learned it. It remains stored in your record, to be searched for as in a library, and used in the necessary moment.

"You, by thinking in this last form, have known what we call the mechanical defense. You must think in order to act, and you separate the senses, the brain, the nerve conduit, and the muscles; all remain independent beings. This is a necessary step in your learning.

"If you meditate on it you will see that when you were born and came to know your environment, first you observed how to act, and then you acted. Yet from this stage you no longer have memories, and that is good for you.

"Now this mechanical stage can serve as a strong defense, but it is slow and difficult in its application, even though every student must live it in the beginning.

"If you have been diligent in your study of the Art, you will see that this stimulus-action, which has begun to integrate itself into your mind, has begun to bear a new fruit. From movement we have reached the mind, which is forced to construct new paths, then to review them in detail. The result of this prepares the student for spontaneity and invisibility.

"The Spontaneous Defense is the next stage. She lives, camouflaged within the previous one, which at the same time never stops growing. When we speak of spontaneity, it is because we have reached a state where the mind has acquired the movement, has made it a part of itself. Just as you once acquired language, with its sound, its hardness or softness, its sweetness or aggressiveness, its closed or open tones that have come to form a part of yourself, inevitably determining something within you, in this same way can Boabom start to become a part of you.

"In this stage you no longer need to reason in order to achieve each of its applications and systems of movement. If you try to remember, you will notice that you lived this process when you felt those bullies grab and assault you. First, you used the mechanical defense and had good results. You did not, however, expect that someone would grab you from behind; that surprised you and you thought. There was doubt, but then you relaxed, and from this was born the spontaneity. Quickly and easily you then dispensed with the other two bullies.

"You shall learn that spontaneity is linked to relaxation and trust: if you are relaxed and believe in the Art, it manifests on its own, perfect and precise. As it is said, it shall be given the opportunity to be born. If you doubt, if you do not trust and therefore you are tense, simple application can be wrong . . . without a spark! This makes it easy for the doubtful and lazy actor to blame the method and not himself. In Boabom, the actor is the method.

"The two positive elements, relaxation and trust, shall be present from the beginning. In any other manner, any alternative of study to Boabom is stillborn. It will only be a waste of time.

"It is normal that in the beginning you cannot feel all of these in a strong way, since it is like a language that is learned, needing its time of mechanics before you can think of it spontaneously.

"In Boabom you will see that spontaneity is born after mechanics, and that one day it simply overcomes them. Remember: your trust in the Art is the mother of your spontaneity, but this process does not stop there. If the student has a profound fidelity toward Boabom, she feels it to her core, living it in all its forms. She will feel how the invisible is born and experience the Inner power in all its splendor.

"The Inner Power is the last step of all these stages. We may also call it invisible or magnetic, for it manifests itself as a field of protection around you that you cannot see or measure. We can also call it a telepathic defense, for it can be noticed by any sensitive being and therefore is transmitted from mind to mind. From another perspective, we can call it a vortex, for its manifestation can be compared to waves or lines of energy. Lastly, we name it simply continuous lucidity, for through its development you must first have a fine, clear, and detailed perception of yourself and the world surrounding you, and second, this lucidity can be produced without stopping, whether you are in a state of being awake or in the dimension of dreams.

"This, which we have called Inner Power, in all its forms, lies latent within the previous stages, ready to be cultivated and awakened. Every being has it.

"Now you will be able to understand why I say that Boabom goes from movement to Inner Power. Each movement has been realized as a technique or special coordination, which in a unique way begins to stimulate certain specific zones of the brain and its roots, the nerves, which together form a whole. From here is born the invisible defense, which is a true shell surrounding your whole body, an aura full of vitality that sprouts through all your organs and forms a harmonious fabric with yourself. And though it might sound surprising, this field can be fed and cultivated.

"Now, with reason can I tell you that this defense is the best of them all. It could happen but once in your lifetime that you should suffer a situation in which your body might be endangered and you must defend it with skill; every day of your life, however, you will face negative energies that can oppose your mind or that simply want to disturb it, influence it, or control it. These negative and invisible emanations can be manifested in simple details: in a disdainful glance, a comment, prejudices imposed in a low voice, or in a simple aggressive gesture. This can happen on many occasions in your life, and the magnetic is really a necessary defense so that your mind can maintain its balance and not be affected by these changes and external negative emanations.

"You shall know also that those who can use this stage with skill can also annul the aggressiveness that surrounds them, whatever its level, without needing to move a finger. This is what you have seen me do with those bandits: they simply sensed my energy, and immediately, instinctively, they knew that it was better for them to run than to continue their confrontation. But the real merits of this energy are focused toward you.

"The birth of this invisibility—of the Inner Power—is the beginning of the end of fear. The inquisitor dies and you are born. But remember that it is a force that feeds from your own rectitude. When the trunk is full of health, its branches are strong and its fruits are sweet and beautiful, without adornments."

Tara was left meditative. She felt that the words of her Guide had resolved many of the things that had happened recently. After a moment of silence, she spoke again to Nnu-Suto. "Your explanation has been extraordinary and surprising, and I think I understand what happened. Will I ever be able to learn to so profoundly develop the Inner Power?"

The pilgrim smiled as he answered. "Of course! If you have been attentive, you will recall how I just now told you that each stage is linked with the others, and therefore all of them are within you now! Through our Art and its paths, one stage feeds another, revives it. If you are persistent and confident, you will see the invisible magnetic field grow around you, just as the Inner Power will grow in your roots . . . as your Art grows."

THAT AFTERNOON was extraordinary for the student; she had much to meditate about. As she advanced, new and incredible surprises opened up for her. She wished only to continue learning from Boabom: day after day she felt, with more strength, that she had been born for it.

Chapter 7

MOON RAY

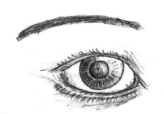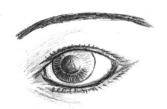

You cannot hope to breathe
without affecting the world.

—*from* The Memories of the Mmulargan

THE GREAT NOCTURNAL STAR shone still in the lonely mountain night. Meanwhile, Tara watched, smiling and silent, from
one of the doors of her house, quietly meditating on the words and
Art of Nnu-Suto.

Meanwhile, her mother was preparing a meal while her sisters
performed some of the household chores. She could hear them tit-
tering about their upcoming marriages, for they would soon marry
two brothers from the village; in this way they entertained themselves. While they spoke, their mother wondered what would become of her eldest daughter, and how it could be possible that the
younger would marry while the elder did not. This was not right, not
according to the traditions. Despite these worries, she had noticed
her daughter in such good spirits of late that she was able to overcome her concerns for her.

Their father remained bedridden, resting from the wound he
had received from the encounter with the bandits. At one moment
he called to Tara, who came immediately to his bed.

"How are you feeling, Father? Can I help you with something?"
she asked attentively.

The old man, a large bandage over one side of his head, replied,
"Daughter, daughter . . . you do not know how comforting your

company is to me. I have been told what happened, and I want you to know that I am proud of you."

"Please, Father, there is no need for you to say that."

"I wanted to tell you that; you need to know. You have always been respectful to me yet at the same time reserved. Somehow I sensed that you were sad. But in this last season you have begun to reflect something different. You look healthier and happier, and you are always positive, lending your energy to others. For one part this has surprised me, for you have changed since you began your lessons with Nnu-Suto."

"It is not so much, Father," she replied. "Only that I feel better, and more relaxed."

"No, no, daughter, it is not that," her father answered, smiling. "You have changed, and I am happy with that change. I am aware that your mother is more apprehensive than I, but she agrees with me. Your sisters, on the other hand, are preoccupied with their marriages, and if they say silly things, please pay them no mind."

"What do you mean?" asked Tara, surprised.

Her father seemed pensive for a few minutes before he spoke again. "This is a small town, my daughter, and unfortunately the intelligence of its speech is related to its size. Many people saw what happened the other day, and many of them are more scared now of you and Nnu-Suto than they were of the bandits that attacked us."

"But that is ridiculous!" She was upset.

"Listen, daughter," her father responded in an understanding tone, taking her hand, "I know this town: everyone is afraid of someone or something different, that some of their neighbors might stand out or break the rules. If this were to happen, it would prove to them how plain and gray their existences really are, just rubbing it in their faces. Now you are a woman who has been an adult for a while now, and you are supposed to marry before your sisters; however, no man from this village interests you, and those who have come close, or whom we have proposed, you have rejected. Besides, as a woman, too, you should be submissive." Tara frowned as he continued. "Do not become upset by this, only listen to me. Many people here look with distrust at someone who was able to stop those fools of the other day."

Tara interrupted him, her tone serious.

"But I do not understand. No one was doing anything—especially the men! Only you, who are now old, acted . . . and naturally I defended you. Would they all prefer that you had died before they saw a woman who was as strong or stronger than all of them?" She sighed. "And what do the women say? After all, we risked ourselves to protect them."

"Worst of all, Tara, is that the same women whom I defended, and whom you too defended by protecting me, are the ones who are talking the loudest. The men, those who were watching and did not dare to act, support the women, speaking not only against you but also against Nnu-Suto."

"But that is not fair, Father. I do not understand," said Tara, while she remembered the rule of Nnu-Suto, to never use the Art. Somehow he seemed to have foreseen the trouble. Her father then continued.

"They claim that he is a wizard, for only a wizard could have the power to stop his attackers in such a way, only such a man could give a woman the power to stop other men as effectively as you did." His tone became sad and angry. "I believe that here the majority are a bit ignorant. But the problem is when the majority become complete idiots! Only a few have defended your attitude and therefore, Nnu-Suto . . ."

Tara's face was downcast. "And what shall I do about it?"

The man answered, caressing her head. "Your father is happy with you and with the way that you are, especially now. I am happy with what you have learned from your teacher. I believe him a good man, but I also believe that this village will never understand, for their heads are too small. If this Nnu-Suto was a real wizard and gave them some amulets—even a dog's tooth would serve to win them! Or if he promised a good harvest or that he would favor their destinies. Or on the other hand, if he threatened them with a hailstorm, I think that everyone would accept him gladly and even pay for his services. I do not know from which world Nnu-Suto comes, but I am afraid that he is not that kind of person. I am afraid that he has wanted only to teach you his Art and nothing else." He added, then, with grief, "Maybe it would be good for him to leave."

This comment saddened Tara deeply. Now that there was something in her life that she truly enjoyed, that gave her energy and vibration, it seemed she would have to let go. She only said: "I know you are right, Father. I might not agree, but I cannot think about myself alone. Anyway, I sense that he will leave soon, for the passes are clear and the weather has become mild enough. I will speak to Nnu-Suto."

THE NEXT AFTERNOON, Tara had her usual lesson. She arrived at the barn a little earlier than usual, but now she was disheartened, not her usual joyful, energetic self. From the distance she could see Nnu-Suto, completely absorbed in his practice. She remained still, so as not to interrupt him.

The old man moved with all the grace and subtlety of a young tree swaying in a soft breeze. The movements of his hands were short and

MOON

RAY

. . .

quick, then soft, wide, and elegant. He turned with grace, and his wide garments beautifully followed the lines of his projections. Sometimes he would use his legs in long steps and unpredictable applications. At the same time he made strange sounds, guttural, deep, and fluctuating as a song made only with melodies born from the breathing tract. His face emanated happiness and surprise and sometimes strength and seriousness.

As she watched him, Tara thought of how much she had yet to learn and how much this man still surprised her. At the same time she remembered the first occasion on which she had seen him and how she had been captivated by Boabom. She thought that, in truth, this teaching was far beyond those flat, unimaginative, and narrow minds. Nnu-Suto should not stay. He was not made for that town; after all, he had described himself as a pilgrim, a lonely wanderer, just like his Art.

When she saw that he had finished, she came slowly closer. They greeted each other with the usual respect, and then the mysterious Guide spoke.

"You have come early to your lessons. You look a bit sad. Tell me what is troubling you."

Not daring to repeat her father's words, she only said, "No . . . nothing."

"When someone says nothing," he replied, "it is usually because it is much."

"Nnu-Suto," Tara said, "I feel that Boabom has done so much good for me, but do you think that people can change?"

The man smiled. "When you say people, you must include yourself, Tara. We are all people, whether we like it or not. The important thing is to feel that, for you, something good has come from what you have learned."

"Of course! I feel better in all ways: I used to easily fall ill; however, now my constitution is much better and I feel strong and healthy. Also, I used to be afraid of everything, but Boabom has made me feel confidence in my own potential. It has made me believe in myself. I feel confident and I like it. Somehow I know it is a sensation that I have always longed for, that for me was an ideal, existing only in the mind, but your Art has made this dream of mine into a reality." After a pause, she continued. "But is it because of the Art or not?"

The pilgrim smiled again. "You must remember that Boabom, more than a determined technique, more than a method, is an energy, something that is transmitted. Invisible, it goes from Guide to apprentice through its movements. This energy, or current, has only one apparent objective, which is the improvement and vitality of the body, yet it has a higher objective as well, which is the mind itself. I used the word 'apparent' because body is also mind: they are inseparable one from the other. It being so, each stage that you have lived within this teaching has affected one as much as the other.

"Before knowing this Way, you were thrown into a monotony that had no solution. Within it there was a constant, imaginary conflict between body and mind, or, more specifically, between what your body felt, your interior mind felt, and what your external thoughts demanded. Boabom, as I have explained on more than one occasion, created an action through each of its movements, and with that has caused a reaction of vitality throughout your physical system. With this we create an order in your metabolism. It is the first way to come closer to the balance that we have named.

"The breathing technique, the stretching systems, and the different projections form part of a framework that has awakened in you, little by little, an energy field or Inner Power, remember? But you must also know that this field is the consequence of your whole body functioning well and in balance. It is the result, which includes body and mind, mind and body, for at last you will discover that they are one and inseparable. Thus we have finally touched the center of ourselves through the consciousness of our own bodies.

"Finally, this aura that now surrounds you, which was always there, though in a lower state, manifests itself slowly as full of strength and splendor, but only because you have earned it by cultivating yourself with discipline and effort. Your body celebrates because it is flourishing and full of life, thanks to the care and nourishment that Boabom has been delivering to it. Being positive, thinking positively, and living full of joy, imagination, dreams, and laughter, these are the greatest achievements of our Arts, for Boabom is an Art for our lives, to give life to life!"

The younger one smiled and could not help but catch the positive energy that the pilgrim emanated. After considering it all, Tara again asked her question. "Noble Nnu-Suto, do you think that this positive energy can change the world?"

The man laughed openly at the question and began dancing, making curious twists of his body. Tara watched and laughed, catching his happiness. After a few moments, he answered. "It has already changed! It has already changed!"

She stared at him, doubtful. He continued. "Tara . . . have you not changed? Were you not a young woman with your head cast down, as you have said yourself? If now you feel full of energy and well with yourself, has not the world already changed? If not, then tell me who the world is?"

The student was left thinking about these words, and she realized that in truth Nnu-Suto was right. She could not, however, help but try to clarify her one remaining doubt. "But, well . . . what I meant was, if others could change with this energy?"

"Tara, Tara . . . who are the others? Are not you the others of the others?" After a brief pause Nnu-Suto added, understanding, "Nevertheless, I know what you mean, but you shall know that the benefits of this Art are reflected in you, toward the exterior world, like a ray from the moon, as the light of the sun is reflected in the moon, enlightening the dark nights.

"This positive energy is transmitted! This is as natural as it is inevitable. Tell me if you do not prefer the company of someone happy and positive rather than one who is bitter and grumpy! Tell me if not many who claim to be religious and spiritual show themselves to be sad or tense, and that better than them you prefer the smile of someone common who does not boast of spiritual superiority. What I mean is that if you achieve this positive aura of the Art and know how to conduct it, the people who surround you will thank you. Somehow you will be changing the world. As a matter of fact, if you have a positive change, you evolve, and with this change alone it is enough to say that the world is changing, evolving."

She smiled and looked at him, yet as she did this, the pilgrim noticed a subtle nostalgia in the eyes of the young woman. He spoke again. "I know that there is much envy, too, much ignorance, that many people resist in the face of the positive, for they see it as a risk, and spontaneously think, 'Why so much joy? What does she want? What does she want from me? If life is so sad, hard, and full of disgrace, why does she speak of the positive?' Or they will say, if they see that you are 'too confident'—he imitated a low, curious voice, adding, "'Why is she so confident? She must be crazy. No one is so confident. Besides, sadness is better, for it lasts longer.' Ahahahaha-hahaha . . ."

Tara and her Guide laughed aloud as he said this. When they stopped laughing, he continued. "You must also consider that every change creates a resistance. It is our natural instinct of survival, of staying with what is familiar, regardless of whether it is good or bad. It is the familiar, so let us speak of it no more. Few are they who dare to experiment, opening new paths; as few are they who dare tread on them for the first time. More than one has been persecuted for that daring. The majority wishes only to remain with what they have seen, with what is documented and certified. But I shall tell you that life is not documented, and that, on the one hand, tradition takes for granted that certain customs are appropriate, but on the other hand, those same traditions were formed by breaking those that came before. Every tradition is also an experiment whose origin we have lost. They are given us readymade. But the time always comes to experiment, to risk something new, even though it sounds new only because we do not know it. Without this there is no evolution, no change, no movement. So do not be surprised by the attitude of people who are afraid of what is different or extraordinary. I know it is hard to face this, and for it you must remember how, one day, I warned you neither to show nor to teach what I was about to transmit to you, for you were the one who wanted to run that risk—not all the rest of the world. But do not worry. Now, enjoy your achievements fully, and if you are happy with yourself, you will see that sooner or later this happiness you possess will become a contagious disease! Hehehe . . ."

Tara laughed, relieved by her teacher's words. For the moment, she forgot that, as her father had said, perhaps it would be good for Nnu-Suto to continue his pilgrimage, that it was now the right time.

After their conversation, they prepared for their afternoon's Boabom class. As always, it was a class full of energy and devotion.

Each movement had been perfected by the student, who showed how attentive she had been as she radiated the ardor she felt for the teaching.

Once the class had finished, and after their moment of meditation, Nnu-Suto closed the class with a comment. "Well, Tara, you have walked a long road this winter. You have advanced enough to obtain your first accomplishment. Our next class will be the last." These words fell as a sentence upon Tara. She felt that somehow her wise Guide had read her mind and knew all that was happening in the village. Nnu-Suto continued, "I will wait for you here the day after tomorrow, but on that occasion we will have a special class in which you will show me everything that you have learned in this time, and I will share with you my last teaching, the finest of them all. I only need you to come willingly, as usual, and to bring a candle. This final lesson will be our way to close this cycle; I will leave the next day, for everything is ready for me to continue on my road. It has been a pleasure to have you as a student."

The young woman could think of nothing to say; she only listened in silence. She felt happy to know that her Guide thought her ready to complete a cycle in the Art, but she felt terribly sad to hear that he was leaving. She knew that it was inevitable, and knowing the determination and strong character of Nnu-Suto, anything she might say would be useless.

Finally, they said farewell as ceremoniously as they usually did. She left, thinking.

Chapter 8

THE CODE OF THE ART

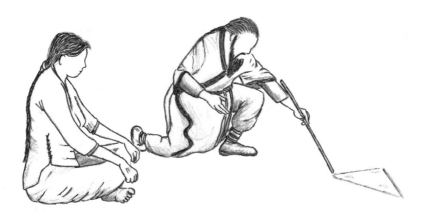

There are three types of search, fed by their own form:
curiosity, knowledge, and understanding of oneself. . . .
The first is strong in its conception but weak in is arrival;
the second is disciplined in its beginning, but limited in its goal;
only the third and final of these forms has neither beginning nor end. . . .
And only this third is identified with the Code of the Art.

—*Subam-Na, "The Voice of the Council,"*
from The Legend of the Mmulmmat II

IN THE BLINK of an eye for Tara, the day on which they would gather for the special class, in which that cycle of teaching would end, had arrived.

Nnu-Suto sat quietly and seemed to be absorbed in the thoughts of a far-off place: perhaps he was recalling that Valley of the Warm Breeze from where, he once said, his teaching came.

The young student gave the proper greeting, then handed him a small basket as a gift. "I have brought you some extra food from my family and me," she said. "Also, there is a cake inside. I hope you like it, for I made it with lots of energy! And here is the candle that you asked for."

The teacher accepted the presents and replied thankfully.

"You are very kind, Tara. You always come with something extra to give. I am happy that I gave you my teachings over this time. But now relax, sit, and tell me, how is your father?"

"He is fine. Your remedy has made him well, and he is already standing and doing a few things."

"I am glad to hear that. Good. Now, listen to what I shall explain before this final lesson." She made herself comfortable, and the pilgrim continued, with tranquility. "We have traveled a long road, full of surprises for both of us. I came to this village driven by the winds, with

no intention of teaching my Art. Life, however, always gives us surprises, and even though our intentions might try to organize our future
and actions, a time comes in which they are overcome by reality. And
this is good! I should have continued on my path without a trace of
passing by here, but something diverted me to this village. Now when
I see you, I understand what it was. I know that this teaching has been
fruitful in you, that it has produced a positive change, and for that I
feel satisfied. You shall know, however, that Boabom is an Art that develops not only physical energy but internal energy as well: I am sure
you have understood this. But this energy manifests itself, showing
you a reality of yourself and an order that is as invisible as it is inevitable. It is about this that I wish to speak with you today, about this
order, which we call the Code of the Art."

Tara felt glad that Nnu-Suto had the confidence to speak of this
with her. While meditating about it, the Guide lit the candle from a
small fire he had built in the corner. Then, taking a stick, he drew a
triangle in the ground, with one of its angles pointing toward them.
In the middle of it, he placed the candle.

"What do the drawing and the candle mean?" asked Tara. "Is it
related to what you have just said?"

"Of course," said Nnu-Suto, smiling. "What you see here is the
Code of the Art, which you can look upon as a figure that is a sign,
a language, an idea, an energy, a movement, which is translated in
three simple and fundamental words from which, with time, three
ideas are born."

In that moment he drew three strange symbols in the angles of
the triangle. The student was completely silent: she did not want
even to breathe, for fear of interrupting the explanation.

The old man continued. "Body, Mind, Art . . . these three elements are inseparable, inevitable, undeniable in their essence: their

work is continuous, unified, and is developed in each self in a constant learning. Pay attention and meditate on this, for this is the Movement. Today you can understand me, and I have been able to transmit Boabom to you because of these three elements, which work in conjunction." Nnu-Suto raised his gaze up high for a second, and then continued. "If you are observant, you will see that what I am explaining is manifested in everything, in one way or another; it is our choice what consequence will produce the interaction of these principles.

"Body . . . the base of everything. Thanks to physical existence, even though not sustained by itself, you and I can speak and communicate in this moment. We exist; a body encourages us in all our reactions, actions, desires, and goals. Our curiosity and thoughts are sustained within it, and this is certainly inevitable; for this reason we must not devalue it, instead giving it care, warmth, and harmony. From this physical base the second manifestation is inseparable, its spontaneous and united consequence:

"Mind . . . she is the ephemeral plasma of the candle, which in its ardor is volatized and lives in continuous change, tied to its base, the body. One is the consequence of the other, and as I have said before, the two are inseparable. This manifestation, based on the physical element, is what brought you to me, to my teaching. Call it reason, thought, ideas, or intelligence, call it feelings, passion, desire, or intuition . . . it is all the same. But because this effect or consequence can be produced by the living spark, at the same instant, simultaneously is generated the last of these three essential elements:

"Art . . . the line. Every living being possesses its own art, and in the end every existence has it. Sometimes these arts are indecipherable but not because they do not exist. It is just that they are far from our understanding, from the art we have generated for ourselves. The mountains have their art. The river has it. . . . The tree in its silent growth, and insects both possess it. Each one of the animals—from all these manifestations you can learn Art . . . the Form, the Way. Within this constant manifestation that flourishes, lives, and dies around us, we exist—humans, animals who proudly call themselves men, mistaken and vain even in their way of classifying and naming themselves.

"Thus you must understand that everything has an art through which it develops and is manifested; it is consubstantial to existence. So we could not say that Art is greater than Mind, or that Mind is greater than Body, or that this is greater than Art, for the three of them are invariably intertwined and of the same nature. At the same time these are only simple ideas that a mind that believes in words can understand. Meditate on this. Even though you do not understand, a time will come in which you will see this, nothing more, in your own Body-Mind-Art.

"In a continuous universal manifestation is born Boabom, our Art, and a noble form by which to develop this inevitable movement. A channel, a path, a way to be walked through self-awareness of the body and its manifestations, freely, without attachment, just as I have shown them to you." Nnu-Suto took that moment to draw again, this time placing new strange figures along the outside of each line of the triangle he had made on the floor, before continuing. "Boabom itself teaches you three new elements that seal the Code. These elements are consubstantial to it, and therefore inevitable in its manifestation. Whether you like it or not, whosoever follows it will live its Code: Discipline, Respect, and Humility.

"Discipline . . . is the idea of will, patience, and constancy, of order, observation, through time, of the teaching that you have begun to walk and therefore to make a part of yourself. It is the key element that you used to come to know and begin your teaching. For any accomplishment you wish to attain in Boabom, discipline is necessary; it is impossible to discover Boabom's effects over time without it. The course of a river does not change just because it flooded one winter: it is constant flooding and changes of its banks that bring it, finally, to a new course, running through different landscapes. So, only with discipline will you be able to live the energy contained in this teaching. In any other way, you would only be fooling yourself.

"You will see, on the other hand, that discipline is manifested in every thing, that any achievement of your existence or of the existence of any being requires discipline, both to build itself and to be lost—these being two extreme stages in a continuous movement, and therefore, change. Alongside this element, at the same time a consequence of it, comes the second element.

"Respect . . . responsibility, values, tolerance. This is a manifestation of trust toward the new road you are beginning to walk. It is the only way to develop this path and, therefore, to continue it. If you do not respect what you are learning, you cannot understand it, cannot harvest its truest, deepest profit. If Boabom is not studied with this element, it will be born false in its effects, incomplete. In the end you will come to the wrong idea of what it really is. When you began, you were full of curiosity, with a clean mind: the natural respect that you showed allowed me to teach you, to open my teaching to you. If it were not this way, I would never have taught you, and this Art would simply not exist for you.

"Lastly, then, and in union as well with all the previous elements, we have the third:

"Humility . . . a synonym for yielding, strength, and clarity of goals. This knowledge will be born or developed within you through Boabom. In the first sense, it will allow you to understand these teachings, for it is thanks to this that you can be receptive to learning. How many people do you know in the world who believe that they know everything! If you thought this way, you could never have learned—you would only revolve around your own limits. If you apply humility, you learn. Thus the one who seems to lose, wins at last, and the one who seems to triumph, is lost in the end.

"Remember your beginnings, Tara, when you asked for these teachings. I treated you badly, I laughed at you, I placed conditions on your learning. However, you remained humble—transmitting those simple words and your own pride—and let yourself be carried by your feeling. This opened the doors of Boabom to you and has let it grow strong within you.

"Thus, through humility you will be able to practice the real strength of these teachings. Boabom is an Art for life . . . to emanate internal and external joy, to be simple, and learn how to enjoy from the simple. Acquiring this for yourself and for your personal Art, you will learn the real dimension of the teachings that have been transmitted to you. This is the Code of the Art, the Code of Boabom."

As he said these words, the wise Nnu-Suto drew a circle within the triangle, around the candle, and when finished, the pilgrim Guide stood. The young woman was left in meditation for a few moments, and thought to herself that she had truly made a good decision to follow the teachings of Nnu-Suto. The truth was that this was a wise man, and he knew of what he spoke. In that moment he indicated to her that she should stand a few steps from his drawing. After making a gesture with their united hands in what seemed like a greeting, he spoke. "Well, Tara, your moment has come: we will review every single one of the movements we have seen, and with that we will close this cycle. You will be free in your path."

She stood, silent and attentive. The last class began. It felt a cli-

THE

CODE

OF THE

ART

. . .

max to all the previous ones. Tara was an extraordinary student, and though it had been hard, in the beginning, for her to understand the movements, one could see clearly that she understood the Code of the Art even before it had been described to her. Her natural discipline, respect, and humility toward the Art had already brought their effect: her movements were full of energy and elegance. The Guide dictated the movements as a soft canticle mantra, and the student did them without difficulty. Positions, breathing, projections, steps, legs, reactions—every stage seemed a harmonic and elegant fabric woven with beauty and strength. It was the living Art, reborn again in a new student.

When they had finished, they sat facing each other in a meditation that reviewed every moment since Tara's first encounter with Boabom: the tests she had to live; the stages she had to overcome and the time she had to stretch to be able to dedicate herself to this teaching; the adventures she had known, the values and work; and finally, the fruit of the last moment. She felt quiet, satisfied . . . but restless.

After a moment the Guide moved toward the drawing and the candle, kneeled with his right knee on the floor, leaving the left to touch his heart. Facing the drawing, he blew out the candle and blew too over the drawing that surrounded it. The air from his mouth joined with a soft breeze that blew from the mountain, and together these forces dissolved that drawing of the Code, erasing it from that place and sending its imaginary lines to the eight winds.

Both of them stood, and before they said good-bye, Tara, who could not help herself, spoke, her voice a bit shaken.

"Are you leaving tomorrow?"

"Yes, Tara, you know already. I must continue my path."

"Have you not considered staying? We could help you settle

here; count on me! I know my family would also help support you," she replied, with hope.

"Boabom is a wandering Art—a nomad—and I am the same. I am sorry, Tara, but I will not stay."

She felt sad. "At what time are you leaving?"

"Tomorrow at dawn, with the sunrise. I will leave by the west road."

"I will be there to say good-bye," Tara replied. "I will bring you some food."

Both then said farewell, and the young woman left.

THAT NIGHT was long for Tara: the light from her candles went out late in her house. Finally, the night made its inexorable advance.

In another house in the village, there was a soft whispering of voices. Nnu-Suto had awakened a few hours before sunrise and was preparing to leave. The wife of the house, who had settled the stranger for the season, heard him rise earlier than she thought he would, and she walked toward his cabin to say good-bye. He had been a good neighbor that winter, and most of all, he had always paid in advance. The lady said: "I suppose you said good-bye to Tara. Did she know you were leaving at this time?"

He answered kindly. "It is better if I leave now, for now the time is right, and it is best that I not waste it. I have a long walk ahead of me. Please, say farewell to Tara and her family for me."

The woman looked at him with a little nostalgia and said good-bye with reverence. She had never come to understand the strange visitor, but despite what people said, she did come to appreciate and respect him.

Nnu-Suto began walking quietly. It was a still night. As he left the village, he turned to look back for one last time. As he gazed up at the starry sky, he made a gesture of respect, joining his two hands. Slowly he started to walk away, but through the opposite path: to the east.

There was a cold breeze that one could feel deep in the lungs. All seemed lonely and silent. After a short while, however, as the road began to slowly go uphill, he was surprised by a familiar voice coming from behind some rocks beside the path.

"Nnu-Suto! Nnu-Suto! It's me. . . ."

The pilgrim turned and smiled: he recognized Tara's voice immediately. Surprised, he replied, "But what are you doing here, Tara?"

"Better I ask what you are doing here? You said you were leaving after sunrise and that you would take the westerly path . . ."

The man smiled. "Well, you know, I changed my mind. Besides, young woman, I do not believe in farewell. Hehehe. Now tell me, what are you doing here?"

"I was waiting for you."

"But here? On the east side and so long before dawn?"

Tara's reply was confident. "You taught me that the Art was surprising, that one must expect the unexpected, and that it is always good to be one step ahead. I knew intuitively that, since you think in that way, you would go not by the west but by the east, and that of course you would leave early. And here I am!" With resolution and joy, she added, "I am leaving with you!"

"With me? Come on, Tara. That cannot happen. No . . . no . . . no . . . Besides, you have your family, and they will be upset. Remember that I told them I would leave in peace. This is not a good expression of peace. . . ."

At that moment another shadow appeared from behind the rock where Tara had been. When the shadow was close enough, Nnu-

Suto heard a low voice. "It is me, Pilgrim, Tara's father . . . and I have come at my daughter's request, for she said that you would accept her only if we were at peace." Nnu-Suto was shocked and left dumbfounded, something that rarely happened to him. "I have come to tell you that she has our support. I have done many stupid things throughout my life, and I do not have the courage to judge my daughter for her decision. Therefore, she can do whatever she wants with her life. She has my consent and my wife's—who was actually quite hard to convince! But anyway, leave in peace. If you happen to come by here again, you will have a home awaiting you."

He then took something from within his clothes: it was an object wrapped in a handkerchief. Giving it to Nnu-Suto, he said, "Please accept this. It is not my idea of a dowry, but let it be a present from the heart. What is wrapped within was made of a rare metal: I inherited it from my ancestors, and I am certain that you will know how to value it." His eyes were full of tears, his voice was shaking. "Now I leave . . . and I leave you free. I will always remember you."

The man approached Nnu-Suto and embraced him with affection; he then embraced his daughter, smiled at her, whispered something in her ear and left, walking with heavy steps and in silence.

The pilgrim remained in silence, too, holding the present in his hands. Seeing that this was a serious matter, he spoke again to Tara. "Are you sure?"

At this she nodded, without a word. He tried again to discourage her, "If you want to follow me . . . better return to your home. . . . I cannot offer you anything. I possess no animals but myself; I have no weapon, no fortune, no gods. . . ." Tara looked him in the eyes, and in that look he could read the strength of her determination.

The pilgrim Guide knew that she had decided that she would follow him, one way or another. Finally he spoke again. "But if you want to walk this way—neither behind me nor in front of me but side by side—of course you are welcome, Tara!"

She embraced him and felt that she could finally rest. Somehow her life had become complete.

THE SUN rose ahead of them, slowly, as it does in the mountains. Two lonely figures were disappearing into the horizon. From afar, their words and laughter could be heard, softly blending with the melody of the breeze and a far-off creek.

"Noble Nnu-Suto, do you think I can have a special name within the Art? Because I have noticed, from what you have taught me, your own name is related to the language of the movements of Boabom."

The pilgrim smiled. "Mmm . . . from your character and the way you show yourself in the Art, you should be named Akimma. . . ."

Curious, she asked: "Akimma? Mmm . . . I like it . . . but what does it mean?"

"Eeeiii! Hehehe . . . I will tell you soon," was the presumptuous answer of the no longer lonely pilgrim.

After a time continuing to walk and laugh, he felt curious about a loose end, so he asked his companion and Apprentice. "I am curious. . . . What if I had left not by the easterly pass but by the west? What would you have done?"

Akimma immediately answered. "Eeeiii!!! Hihihihi . . ." Behind her laughter, Nnu-Suto's laughter spontaneously echoed, as he thought to himself that she would be an exceptional student.

· · ·

FEW NOW remember these successes.

Those who still remember say that perhaps they traveled to a dimension outside time and the understanding of men. Others said that they saw them fading into the high passes of far mountains; others are sure that they crossed through certain hidden caves that took them to the lost Valley of the Warm Breeze. Some even say that they continued to teach in other villages. No one is certain. But what everyone says is that Tara's father definitively forgot his taste for fermented drinks, and some even saw him doing strange movements and breathing in ways that they believe he learned by secretly imitating his daughter. Even more, it is said that he taught these basic movements to his wife and two other daughters, who finally learned to respect and truly value him.

Second Step

THE ART

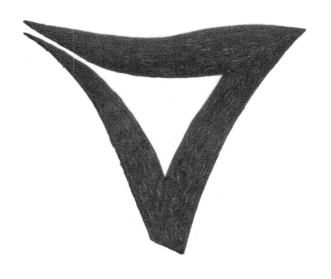
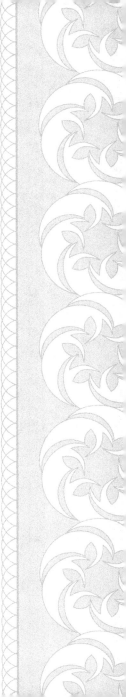

Chapter 1

Walking from Theory to Practice

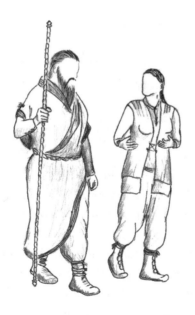

A good wheel appreciates being spun.

—*Amsei Fadis, from* The Legend of the Mmulmmat

FROM THE TALES of Boabom to actual reality is only one step, and it is this that we are going to give you now.

Though they may sound surprising, facts that may seem extraordinary happen every single day. Each individual must be able first to distinguish them, then to live them or not. This book, in its First Step, develops a short story about the Art and its Way. Perhaps this story, compared with reality, may not be literal, but be sure that its essence has been preserved, and the facts upon which I have based it are even more surprising. At the same time I have tried, through this story, to give you a practical idea of what this teaching is about, its general form, and the essential principles that give it energy and breath, not only as an Art but as a way of life. There is much to be read between the lines: I leave that to you.

The idea too is for you to have understood, bit by bit, how the Art would be developed practically, how real students learn it and move through its basic stages and accomplishments. Each of the eight previous chapters is related to the teachings of the technical stages of the Art: they complement one another and are woven together. The Second Step, the Art, is destined to transmit to you the basis of this teaching, which will require both your physical and mental senses. This introduction will first explain the antecedent elements that must be considered, then more fully develop the technique itself. The chapters following this one will explain the movements themselves, how they are coordinated and applied, and how they must be executed in order for them to have a real effect on your personal development.

This section is an opportunity for you to dive in and live your own story, the one you will write as a student of the Boabom School. Now it is your turn. The Inner Power is there in everyone: it depends only on you to awaken it!

Maybe the words Inner Power sound over the top, or that speaking of extraordinary effects in both your physical and mental energy is easy to say but not real. Healthy skepticism is valid, and from that point of view our teachings also say that one must speak with facts: this is the least you can ask of any claim we might make. As evidence behind my words, in the Third Step of this book you will learn more about the School itself, and the students of both Boabom and Seamm-Jasani speak about their own experience and development in their health, energy, daily life—even their dreams! We accompany this with a meticulous scientific study prepared by a group of professionals who have prepared the first approach to this Art from the perspective of modern science. The facts speak for themselves.

Now, as a student of this ancient Art, you have the opportunity to discover its secrets and to live the benefits of a teaching whose only goal has been and remains to cultivate the vitality of body and mind to its maximum, to develop their essential physical-psychical power, and in that way to live better, longer, and with more intensity: to experience for yourself an integrated system of self-healing through movement.

Through this second stage you will see those movements that correspond to the first steps taken by any beginning Boabom student. An ultimate or higher development of this Art would take years (and *many* books!), for it covers an incredible number of movements and systems, both physical and psychical. This book represents a *simple* and *accessible* way for anyone to begin, with no need for any prior knowledge. As you should appreciate, it is about a long journey, yet every long journey begins with one simple step, and you have already taken it! Now it is time to take the second. The important thing for you as a student-reader is to feel it, and in that way to understand. Walking from theory to practice! If you feel that you have the necessary initial discipline, and with that the seriousness to continue with this step of the book, to take the Art into practice, then read carefully what I am about to explain about how to develop Boabom in yourself . . . and welcome!

A great positive energy—and may you have the greatest of successes in this adventure! The great adventure of Boabom!

The Art of Defense, Meditation, and the Inner Power

Beyond Defense

The first thing you should know before entering into this technique itself is that Boabom is not simply an Art of Defense like so many others, for it goes beyond the purely physical. Its movements are related to channels and nets of energy that, when animated in conjunction with one another and with a positive mind, can awaken an uncommon internal force and an ascending cycle of strengthening health. The energy that we can generate will always surpass logic because that is the reasonable experience (and that, preconceived or culturally inherited) of reality . . . and this energy (for the good of us all!) does not stick to reason: it simply is.

Defense is only the external face of this Art, even though as such it can be and is incredibly effective. But remember that these movements are a tool for your mind, a form to center it, to discipline and focus it. The student must view the technique as a method, not a goal in itself. As it would be said in Sanskrit: the sound of the Boabom breathing would become a meditative mantra, and its path of defense would constitute a metamorphous yantra.

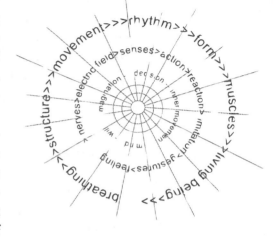

To summarize what has been said previously: Boabom teaches that the body-mind can generate an energy superior to that which is usual, and for this it must work as a net or vortex that feeds back into itself. To achieve this, it is important to emphasize every detail, for all of them are important when taking this Art into practice, whether we take it simply as a form of defense or look deeper inside at the Inner Path of Meditation. The breathing, the structure, the movement, even the thoughts must be seen as a spider web. One thing affects another, and they all must be cultivated and developed simultaneously. When practicing each exercise, each technique or coordination, remember this: insist, and make your whole spider web vibrate . . . the awakening will come in its time.

Understood in this way, Boabom becomes a profound force, conducted through movement, that directly stimulates the subconscious and the hidden psychic energy. I do not intend by this to say you will become some sort of magician, but I do mean that you will be able to achieve something as simple as it is incredible: to live fully, healthy, with confidence and full of vitality, immune to the negative external energies. For a moment you will be able to enjoy the approach to yourself. This is the real goal—the awakening of a new day.

Always keep in your mind that behind one facet, which you may see as defense, is hidden the noble nature of an Art that seeks to increase your vitality while tuning your perception of the world and yourself, nothing more. Parallel to this you will see how many of your illnesses vanish as you become stronger: this is the great power of movement.

About the Inner Power

According to the most common meaning of these words, Power can be interpreted as ability, skill, or capacity, and is a synonym for authority, control, influence, supremacy, and command. If we take the word Inner, we will find it to mean located or occurring within something, or, an example that can aid us, the part of something that is farthest from the edge.

Trying to use these same words and their common meanings, I have aimed for a very simple idea. We have been raised and formed within a particular culture that, in an attempt to let nothing escape from its conventions or conveniences dictated by the prevailing group in a determined historical moment, in the end restricts that ability, skill, or capacity that we all possess, from birth, and that corresponds to us simply by being alive. We can relate that strength and capacity to intelligence, will, creativity, or simply to our physical capacity, but we can also interpret it as an eternal current that sings and vibrates, flowing translucent, clear, and pure, waiting to be discovered. This was born open to everyone, and in that way it shall remain!

If we look for examples, we can easily find one in the obscure Dark Ages. That era was rife with persecution, burning or imprisoning those who showed psychic power or capacity, whether through intelligence, curiosity, or simply extraordinary capacities. Sometimes I wonder how many wise men, and especially how many wise women, were murdered or frustrated in those ages, how much genius was forbidden, how many inventions waited centuries to exist, prohibited by the cultural tendencies of the moment. As well, I wonder how many destructive weapons might not exist today if the construction of warlike toys had not been encouraged, paid for, and celebrated by those same people who were capable of compassionlessly burning a defenseless old woman, accusing her of being a witch simply because she committed the terrible sin of knowing the secrets of some herbs or simply for being the seed of a vision that was different from the one held by the prevailing patriarchy.

I do not intend to bore you with this or to deviate into a critique of history; I only wish to explain that, in one way or another, we have been limited in that natural ability, skill, or capacity, which we all possess, by the culture that surrounds us. Every time someone close to us tells us what or what not to do without any argument or example (meaning: consequence), or if an entire culture doing this with the same weak arguments and examples, we can feel that power languish, die, or even worse, become the servant of the ones firmly in command of the cultural guidelines. I wonder how many scientists nowadays are working salaried in warlike enterprise? When will the day come when the genius ceases to serve the corrupt? As the saying goes: "Good try, poor execution." Although many may think these comments overimpassioned or out of place, I will say that no,

WALKING
FROM
THEORY
TO PRACTICE
. . .

115

in fact, they are directly related to our subject. Every human being represents, in itself, the examples he or she sees in society (and maybe for this, sometimes, we reject it too much), and this discussion should offer a different perspective on how to be and behave.

On the other hand, we have used the word "Inner" for the hidden face that a great part of our energy possesses: this is a great capacity we rarely cultivate, our personal essence, or what we do not show. This part can be developed positively if we can release it from the limits surrounding it. This inner quality is the most feared facet of being: it is the latent self, the yet uncontrolled, or in other words, that which is not normalized. In history, it is the range of what is unpredictable.

Like every energy, this energy can be conducted in a positive way, or it can, in turn, become self-destructive. That it will manifest itself is inevitable, for in one way or another it always does. Sooner or later, nothing escapes movement.

That is why the Awakening of the Inner Power in Boabom can be interpreted as being yourself, knowing yourself free of prejudices, being beyond negative influences and the control of those who tell us not this and not that. Yet at the same time it is a synonym for a great humility, of knowing how to clearly contemplate oneself in every aspect, in order to channel all our internal and external energy in a free, strong, and positive way. Germane to this is the example I gave a few paragraphs before about scientists, for this is about conducting the intellect: first, free from corrupt administration with selfish interests that prevail over the studious, the supposedly intelligent; second, strong enough to know what she can be worth for herself, without relying on flattery or a salary built on the shoulders of innocents; and third, positive, for she must be willing to use all of her genius in unrelenting creativity, as well as in evolution of the self, of humanity, and of the planet, for these three are the same.

To move into another subject, I would like to clarify some Eastern ideas on this subject. In a great part of this Eastern culture, such manifestation or awakening is related to what, in Sanskrit, is called chakra, and about which I made a small pun in my previous book. I hope that the correct meaning of my words has been conveyed and understood, for within Boabom one intends to reach the trunk (or essence of oneself) not only the branches (the chakras). If the trunk is healthy and vital, all else glows, shines, and at the same time loses importance.

This Inner Power announces to you that you *can,* that when you direct and focus your mind, disciplining it in a direct way and with positive motives, you always *can.* Whether it is using our energy in the inventive capacity, in the joy of being alive, or in pure psychic power, the Art of Boabom will be a key method in that development. For that, work with discipline and with your vital, physical element, and with gratitude you will see this answer come to you: the changes will manifest themselves in fine details, like a warm breeze on a wintry mountain. Let the mind be stimulated through every exercise and technique, and with patience, this Inner Power will become a new food, a solid balance between yourself and the external world.

Though it may sound strange, this day you have opened a door to another dimension, one that can transport you to ancient Tibet—the one that has survived beyond empires, the one that has managed to keep its Inner Power intact. Its mysteries and its lost Art have also suffered persecution at the hands of those who are not capable of imposing themselves with arguments. Study it and make it silently tell you its secrets as it awakens in you the latent energy that will revitalize your body and open your mind as never before.

WALKING

FROM

THEORY

TO PRACTICE

. . .

117

Considerations for the Practical Course

Implements

Although it may sound as if I have said this before, I say this again with the same certainty: for this course, you need only your Body-Mind and Art, and nothing else. If you are one of those who likes to collect lots of trash (sorry!)—exercise machines they sell on television—simply forget them, for they are worthless. Even though you can see how they try to justify them with incredible presentation, as tridemensional and repetitive as to make you believe that you need them, do not believe it. Be simple, work directly with your body and mind, for both have been calibrated for thousands of years to act in a natural and optimum way. Do not become one more piece in this modern machinery. Out with the weights, torture beds and chairs, children's balloons from the seventies that have been remastered for exercise, bicycles that go nowhere, and however many things might be invented in the period from now, when I am writing this book, to the day it reaches your hands.

Being very clear on this point, you are ready to begin seriously this study proposed by this second step: the practical Art. You need only follow the basic instructions I will detail below.

Order

If you look at the next two chapters, you will notice that they are fully dedicated to the development of the Art in its two main facets, as well as in a third, which is more coordinative. The first two are always necessary. Take into account that every engine needs to warm itself up to achieve its fullest power, and therefore you need the Boabom Jass-U (second step, chapter 2), which is a simple summary of basic exercises meant to prepare you for the second stage. Once we have delved into and advanced in the first, we can venture into the Osseous Art, or Boabom itself (second step, chapter 3); thus, *never begin the Osseous Art without first warming up.*

Now the first thing to do is to organize your own class. In general, it is said that Boabom is better digested after the body has had some activity, meaning not too early in the morning. In practice, however, this depends largely on one's own habits. More important is that the session should be far from previous meals, so simply look for a stable time within your own schedule. Ideal is to do the class twice a week, for two well executed sessions are enough. If you feel you can give more, add one more session. An example of twice a week would be Mondays and Wednesdays; for three times it could be Mondays, Wednesdays, and Fridays. We always try to put one or two days in between the classes so that we can rest: this serves as a recovery time both for the muscles and the psyche. Think that you need to make each movement a part of yourself, and this requires constancy much more than intensity.

About Seamm-Jasani

Perhaps you have also read my book about Seamm-Jasani. If so, you are one of my old student-readers. If so, or if in the future you acquire that book, you will notice that both Arts are closely related and therefore complement each other perfectly. On the one hand, Seamm-Jasani develops as simple and relaxed exercises and stretch-

WALKING
FROM
THEORY
TO PRACTICE
. . .

119

ing: it is slow, deliberate, and detailed in its development, and its breathing technique is elongated. On the other hand, we have Boabom, which develops the opposite face, for its warmups are fast and strong and the technique itself is quick—executed like a flash or spark—yet at the same time precise, complete, and solid, with a breathing technique that is sharp. Both Arts require dedicated study. A good student in one will find new shades in the other. While perfecting one she will also perfect the other. In fact, you may notice exercises that are practically the same, with only slight differentiations in their execution.

If you can command the basics of both of these facets, Seamm-Jasani and Boabom, you can just review one class of one kind, then one class of the other. A perfect example for a more quiet metabolism would be: Mondays, Seamm-Jasani session; Wednesdays, Boabom session; and Fridays, Seamm-Jasani session. If you consider your metabolism a bit more restless and invigorated, you can organize this in reverse.

As you can see, there are no strict rules, only general guidelines. Each one must look for his or her own identity in the rhythm of learning and practice. Through all of this, however, *do not abuse yourself!* Do not think that repeating these exercises over many hours or repeating them thousands of times will give you better results. Keep always to the medium state: "It is much better a good few (and constant, too!) than many and poor." Anyway, there is another saying that mentions something about starting out a racehorse and ending up a donkey, and another that speaks of the tortoise and the hare, and so on. I am certain you understand.

Pedagogical Method, Class Time, and Intensity

Boabom has a strict evolutionary and pedagogical development, and this is one of its main components: it imitates the steps of life, from crawling to the pure use of mind. A teacher prepared in Boabom has a defined criteria for taking the student step-by-step, according to her or his quality or the general qualities of a group, in order to let him or her learn in a fluid way, not abruptly or brusquely, as so often happens in systems developed by people with mentalities as arrogant as they are ignorant.

Owing to the limitations in the nature of a book, I have tried to compensate for the lack of a teacher with the Pedagogical Chart, which is found at the end of this chapter. The whole of this book is gradually unfolded through it, in a way to ensure that both psychological understanding and physical-vital development go hand-in-hand. Follow it as exactly as you can.

As for the time you should dedicate to each session, you can vary this with the knowledge that you will gain through practice. In general, you can begin with twenty minutes, slowly expand to thirty minutes, and then eventually to a full forty-five minutes once the class has unfolded completely (meaning ten to fifteen minutes of Jass-U plus thirty to thirty-five minutes of Osseous Boabom). At the outset, time will disappear as you try to understand and memorize each exercise; but once you have learned them well, they will take less time. Once you have achieved this and you find yourself executing the initial movements continuously, it will be time to add the others and develop a more complete class. I insist: the main thing is to be patient and very, very conscientious.

As for the intensity of the exercises, try to begin by knowing

WALKING

FROM

THEORY

TO PRACTICE

. . .

121

them in a quiet way. Once you have built a basic confidence, increase the rhythm and power. As this matures in you, the relationship between intensity-rhythm-power should increase, lasting in a balanced way through the whole class. Remember that Boabom is a strong and sharp Art, but that it also requires wisdom to put it into practice.

About the Drawings and Reference Boxes

Please do not say that my drawings are ugly! I am very sensitive on this subject . . . Hehehe. But seriously, now, I know I do not draw perfectly, but the idea is that you are able to understand the central meaning of each exercise. Besides, I have had my special assistant, Amlom, who, as usual, has patiently helped me to finish the drawings as perfectly as possible.

As you will see, the drawings indicate frontal and lateral angles for your better understanding. If any movement does not have many perspectives, it is related to another one that has been previously detailed. Anyway, we prefer to use drawings again, instead of photographs, for they are easier to understand, and can, in just a few lines, show ideas, not to mention a bit of poetry—and what is an Art without a bit of poetry?

In some cases we have added notes on Common Mistakes, illustrated with simple drawings. This shows how *not* to do the exercise, or wrong positions into which one can easily fall when doing the movement.

For each exercise and technique you will also see that, for the sake of clarity, I have annexed a special Reference Box to serve as a summary of each movement, so that in the future you will be able to skip the detailed explanation given for each exercise and go directly to this box for reference. In this box are also mentioned the muscles affected by some of the movements, only for curiosity and general reference, as the purpose of this book is not a detailed anatomical analysis of these movements; for that would be quite a long and complex task, considering that only one movement can involve many muscles at the same time, each different in its intensity and form. Imagine, it is said, that for one vocal sound more than fifty muscles move! In this Art, the example holds true: the body and mind in concert, together generating an energy that cannot be coldly digested or compartmentalized.

For ease of understanding, each item in the Reference Boxes is shown in the following format:

Second Step: Chapter 2. Boabom Jass-U, or The Art of Osseous Awakening

Symbolic Name: Simple metaphorical designation of the exercise.

Initial Position: Form in which the body must be just before beginning the exercise.

Breathing: Application of the breathing technique for the specified exercise.

Affected Muscles: General description of the muscles or area directly affected by the movement.

Duration: Time spent on the exercise, whether in seconds or number of repetitions.

Degree of Difficulty: Quick classification from 1 to 5 of the difficulty level of the particular exercise; 1 is the simplest, 5 the most complex.

Remember that if you have any physical limitations, you should pay close attention to this classification.

Second Step: Chapter 3. Boabom— The Technique of the Osseous Art

Symbolic Name: Designation of the technique, referring directly or metaphorically to its development or objectives.

Initial Position: Form in which the body must be just before beginning the exercise.

Breathing: Application of the breathing technique for the specified exercise.

Duration: Time spent doing the exercise, given as the number of repetitions.

Defense Application or Basic Objectives: General reference to the potential goals of the movement, or the points of application as defense or projection.

Some Advice About Food, Diet, and General Precaution

Remember that Boabom is an Art that demands much, both physically and mentally; therefore, always remember: *Do not eat before your class.* Do not misunderstand me: this does not mean that you should not eat at all, but that you should refrain from heavy meals for about two or three hours before your class. If your sessions are in the morning, this should not be a big problem. But if they are at another time, please be more careful. As for drinking liquids, it is enough to not do so for thirty minutes beforehand, if these are light juices or water. This is for several reasons: first, to begin your exercises with a full stomach is like flying through a storm in a plane loaded with loose suitcases and full of passengers who have not actually fastened their seat belts. Because your stomach has no seat belts to fasten what you eat, it is much better to prevent than to cure, and therefore much better to take your lesson with a relatively empty stomach, for if you do not, the internal walls of your stomach will suffer, and the class will do you more harm than good.

Another reason is that when the digestive system is in the process of absorbing food, it requires more blood than usual. The Art, in its execution, requires a great amount of this precious liquid; thus to avoid such a conflict, avoid eating too close to this exercise. For the same reason it is good to avoid eating right after a session. By eating too soon, we delay the body's recovery, which is based on the circulation of the blood. It is best to wait a short while, instead using the time for a shower or a bath.

As for food in general, feel free to eat what you think you need; Boabom will do the rest. By this I mean that, little by little, you will come to know your own metabolism and needs, and through this you will eat what is right. You will discover your own Middle State. Forget models on TV: real life is much better and simpler than they pretend. Be patient and disciplined in your Art, and it will show you the way.

If you are a vegetarian, continue so; if you are a carnivore, the same. Boabom does not impose rules about eating: it would be too pretentious to say that we have the ideal diet for 6 billion different bodies—or are we more by now? Each organism has its own caloric requirement, its individual necessities, its own alimentary personality, so to speak.

In Boabom we recommend that you begin with the beginning: first, organize the house, clean it profoundly, and then see what it

WALKING

FROM

THEORY

TO PRACTICE

. . .

125

needs, and what is sparing (or was hidden!). Dedicate yourself to the Art in depth, relax, and get to really know yourself, you (and that means you!) . . .

Now if you have a diagnosed disease, please do not forget to speak with your physician. This Art does not work miracles: it will help you if you develop it, but each individual must also take the precautions that his or her body asks, in each individual case. Do not change diets abruptly, only eat well. What you should remember is to drink a lot of liquids, for Boabom, when well executed, can cause you to lose a large amount of liquid in a short time. The ideal is to drink liquids distant from meals but in abundance (around three liters a day is an excellent goal).

Environment and Clothing

As for the proper clothes for this practice, do not worry, just find something comfortable, like normal exercise clothes, preferably cotton. The main point is to feel comfortable doing the movements.

As I mentioned before, for the best, you need the simplest. In fact, try not to use sneakers, but do the class barefoot, which is a more natural and real way to work. If this is not possible, do not worry, as you can accommodate to work with shoes. Just please try to make it some kind of sport shoe.

As for the color of your clothes, again it does not matter: the habit does not make the monk. Even though our school has a certain discipline regarding clothes, this is not prescriptive as it only symbolizes an order. What is important is that you work with this Art and make it come alive in you. Remember that the best clothing is our own skin!

In relation to environment, you will come to see that the development of Boabom does not require much space; perhaps you can do it perfectly in your own room. Just find your own space and get comfortable. The Great Chamber of the Boabom teaching is everywhere: in the countryside, the mountains, a barn, a large room, your own office, or the small living room in your house. You can also look for an outdoor place: if there is a park nearby, it could work perfectly. What is most important is that you feel comfortable; try to pick a place that is more or less quiet, where you won't be interrupted by a large crowd of curious people staring at what you are doing, since Boabom is an Art that calls attention. As I was saying, what is most important is your own tranquility and concentration, and that you feel free to work openly, to develop all of your power and expression with the maximum of energy in your movements and breathing technique, no matter the noise you make! You need to discharge all of your energies in order to refill yourself with energies that are new, clean, and revitalized!

Think positive, and you will see that you will find the best place.

Other Concerns Before and After a Class

Since the development of this Art is very strong, you will see that the first classes, if well executed, can cause some muscular distress, soreness, or cramps. If this happens, do not worry, for this is normal for a student who has executed the techniques with proper emphasis. With time and constancy in the exercises, this soreness will pass. Some areas that are normally affected by this are the backs of the thighs, the stomach, and the arms.

To avoid most of these small discomforts, after a class you can take a hot shower. Try not to let the water be too cool, for you will only con-

WALKING

FROM

THEORY

TO PRACTICE

. . .

127

tract the muscles suddenly, which will only make any cramping worse. Hot water is always the best, as it allows for better blood circulation and therefore a better recovery. If you can take a bath afterward, you may want to add some sea or raw salts, and you will notice that it makes you feel very good. Just do not take too long a bath.

Another important piece of advice is to not wear any jewelry, rings, or other metallic elements during the class. Remember that Boabom has very strong and quick movements; therefore, as a precaution, it is better to avoid any metals. Remember that the best always requires the least materialism: too many adornments only distract us from our real essence. The Art of Boabom is something natural, working with the body-mind in its essence, and like anything natural, an external element only produces a delay in the circulation of energy. If we think about it, who was born with jewels, rings, earrings, or piercings of any kind in their skin or limbs? The answer is obvious.

Trust evolution: for a reason, it has made us what we are, with the adornments we already have. If you wish to try this Art full of bagatelles dangling about you, whether for superstition, sentimentalism, or exhibitionism, such is your free will, but I take no responsibility for the results or possible dangers: it is you who shall take that risk.

In Case of Disease or Physical Challenge

It is also important that you have a medical checkup before beginning the Osseous Art. Be aware that these exercises and techniques have, in general, a very strong and solid development and therefore make certain physical demands on the student. So be cautious. As I always say, "This author (teacher) does not take responsibility for irresponsible people."

Now, with all this in mind, you can begin Boabom. If you have any debilitating disease, the best thing would be to begin with Seamm-Jasani, the gentle stage, and then adapt little by little. After a time working with the Gentle Art, and as you feel more confident, you can begin Boabom on firm footing. People have many kinds of problems, and it would be difficult to give a special solution for each case, but if you are careful and patient, you will see that you can adapt yourself to each movement of Seamm-Jasani and Boabom.

Whatever the way, if you think that you cannot do an exercise or if you feel that it may be too difficult, just continue with the next one. With patience and time you will be able to understand them all, and you will be able to do them by your own measure. Remember: wanting creates doing!

Physical Age Does Not Matter!

This point is very important. Boabom is an Art for everyone. Age, just like the country you come from, what you believe in, or what language you might speak, does not matter: what is important is your energy and your desire to cultivate it.

This Art has never followed the traditional macho point of view of most Eastern cultures (and Western, too!). In the great mountain the woman has at least the same range as the man, and therefore we say that Boabom, from its beginning thousands of years ago, was specifically designed to be cultivated by both the feminine and masculine energy.

In regard to age, it is normal that an older person may need to

WALKING

FROM

THEORY

TO PRACTICE

. . .

129

move more slowly and take the learning process with more tranquility. For this there are two options: first, the student can begin with Seamm-Jasani, which, from a certain point of view, is a gentler Art that is more simple to follow, and then later begin with Boabom. The other solution to soften the development of Boabom would be to simply extend, to double or triple, the length of time suggested in the Pedagogical Chart, and extend the complete process to five or six months instead of three.

As for children, there is no problem either. For them, you can follow the same recommendation as above (to double or triple the time indicated in the Pedagogical Chart), and they can then take fewer classes (once a week, perhaps). In each class they would need only to do the basic movements, not dedicating too much time to them, and as he or she becomes adapted and begins to enjoy and want the class more, you can add new movements and allow more time for each session. The main idea is not to abuse the individual. Children work at a different pace, and thus you cannot tell them exactly what to do, as it will only cause them harm. (And it is terrible to try to make children look like adults; it would be much better, in fact, to have adults imitate children!)

Children can be perfectly taught discipline along with joy, and at the same time with a taste for what they are doing!

The important point is that everyone can!

Pedagogical Chart

Here you will find the Pedagogical Chart, which will indicate, session by session, how to integrate and develop the warm-ups or Jass-U (second step, chapter 2), the Technique of Boabom (second step, chapter 3), and the Forms of Reaction (second step, chapter 4). The first two must be developed slowly, and at the end can be complemented by the third system; thus first you should complete the Jass-U, later the Boabom, and finally the Forms of Reaction. To understand this whole process, you need only follow the chart closely and increase your efforts with the sessions.

Remember that the purpose of this chart is to make this book as similar as possible to the way in which this Art is usually taught, which is step by step. Do not take this book as a catalog of exercises, as too often happens with books related to physical therapies, which usually show a series of positions that have neither a beginning nor an end, nor a fluid progression. It is important that you understand this book as a beginning, which must be studied in a gradual development, yet it is not all there is! Follow the chart precisely: the learning process depends on this, in its ease, pedagogy, and understanding.

This chart organizes the course over three months, in which time you should achieve a certain maturity and a complete development of this book. From that point forward, you can continue perfecting the movements you know or you can look for a Boabom School! The path is always open to the one who really seeks!

If you look at this chart, you will see that the Jass-U is developed quickly, and that after four weeks or a month you should be doing all of those movements without problems. Boabom, on the other hand, grows more slowly and requires more study, concentration, and memory, and thus more time.

All of the warm-up exercises, as well as the techniques themselves, are shown in the order of ideal continuity through a complete class. The check marks on the right side indicate when each movement should be added to the class, while the small arrows show that

WALKING

FROM

THEORY

TO PRACTICE

. . .

131

it is not yet time to do them. In this way, bit by bit, you can complete the class through an adaptation that is slow and whole. Give yourself time for this.

As you may observe, in the technical part you must first study the basic positions. Already, by the second class, these are not reviewed separately but are included within other techniques (for example, the Solid Fist is used in the Double Force of the Spiral, and so on). This is why they are not marked as the classes continue. Also, once the Universal Position has been learned, it will be reviewed two times between every technique, from number six to number fourteen. This will also happen with The Way and The Applied Way, which last only a few weeks before being assimilated in successive coordinative stages (numbers seventeen to twenty-two). All of this is indicated in the chart.

Finally, the Forms of Reaction require more time for maturation and are developed alternatively, near the completion of the three months.

Very likely you will be able to develop all of these movements faster than is indicated in the chart, but the idea is to go step by step and to do your sessions in a continual and consistent manner over time. You will see that you will understand much better, and you will enjoy learning them much, much more.

If you like, you can first read the whole book and then later, in practice, dedicate yourself to studying the movements one at a time, according to the Chart. Or you can simply begin now and see the movements for the first time when the chart requires you to.

Remember, the most important elements are constancy and discipline!

Welcome to Boabom, the Art of One Thousand Ways!

PEDAGOGICAL CHART

Week Number:	1	2	3	4	5	6	7	8	9	10	11	12
Month:	1st Month				2nd Month				3rd Month			

FINISHED CLASS IN ORDER

Part 1. The Art of Awakening

	1	2	3	4	5	6	7	8	9	10	11	12
1. Base Position	✓	Studied within the development of subsequent exercises.										
2. Freeing the Energy	✓	✓	✓	✓	✓	✓	✓	✓	✓	✓	✓	✓
3. The Puppet's Advance	✓	✓	✓	✓	✓	✓	✓	✓	✓	✓	✓	✓
4. The Puppet's Retreat	→	✓	✓	✓	✓	✓	✓	✓	✓	✓	✓	✓
5. Breathing Technique of the Inner Power	✓	✓	✓	✓	✓	✓	✓	✓	✓	✓	✓	✓
6. Harvesting	→	→	→	✓	✓	✓	✓	✓	✓	✓	✓	✓
7. Heel-Hand Game	→	✓	✓	✓	✓	✓	✓	✓	✓	✓	✓	✓
8. Touching the Earth	✓	✓	✓	✓	✓	✓	✓	✓	✓	✓	✓	✓
9. The Pincers	✓	✓	✓	✓	✓	✓	✓	✓	✓	✓	✓	✓
10. The Fists That Hum	✓	✓	✓	✓	✓	✓	✓	✓	✓	✓	✓	✓
11. To Lift and Spill the Ewer	✓	✓	✓	✓	✓	✓	✓	✓	✓	✓	✓	✓
12. Swaying on the Mountain	→	✓	✓	✓	✓	✓	✓	✓	✓	✓	✓	✓
13. Flight of the Butterfly	✓	✓	✓	✓	✓	✓	✓	✓	✓	✓	✓	✓
14. The Embracing Bird	✓	✓	✓	✓	✓	✓	✓	✓	✓	✓	✓	✓
15. The Fish That Rises	→	✓	✓	✓	✓	✓	✓	✓	✓	✓	✓	✓
16. The Flower of the Inner Power	✓	✓	✓	✓	✓	✓	✓	✓	✓	✓	✓	✓
17. The Boabom Fist	✓	✓	✓	✓	✓	✓	✓	✓	✓	✓	✓	✓
18. The Boabom Palm	→	→	✓	✓	✓	✓	✓	✓	✓	✓	✓	✓
Repeat: Freeing the Energy	✓	✓	✓	✓	✓	✓	✓	✓	✓	✓	✓	✓
19. The Balance	→	→	→	✓	✓	✓	✓	✓	✓	✓	✓	✓

PEDAGOGICAL CHART

	Week Number:	1	2	3	4	5	6	7	8	9	10	11	12
	Month:		1st Month				2nd Month				3rd Month		

	1	2	3	4	5	6	7	8	9	10	11	12
20. The Breathing That Closes the Circle	✓	✓	✓	✓	✓	✓	✓	✓	✓	✓	✓	✓

Part 2. Boabom—The Technique of the Osseous Art

INITIAL POSITIONS

	1	2	3	4	5	6	7	8	9	10	11	12	
1. Osseous Field	✓	✓	✓	✓	✓	✓	✓	✓	✓	✓	✓	✓	
2. Normal Position of Balance	✓												Practiced within the techniques themselves.
3. The Solid Fist and The Solid Palm	✓												Practiced within the techniques themselves.
4. The Fist That Is Born and The Palm That Is Born	✓												Practiced within the techniques themselves.
5. Universal Position	✓												This position is used two times (x2) between each technique from 6 to 14.

INITIAL HAND TECHNIQUES

	1	2	3	4	5	6	7	8	9	10	11	12
6. The Force of the Spiral, Middle	✓	✓	✓	✓	✓	✓	✓	✓	✓	✓	✓	✓
7. The Force of the Spiral, Low	→	✓	✓	✓	✓	✓	✓	✓	✓	✓	✓	✓
8. The Force of the Spiral, High	→	→	✓	✓	✓	✓	✓	✓	✓	✓	✓	✓
9. The Force of the Double Spiral	→	→	→	✓	✓	✓	✓	✓	✓	✓	✓	✓
10. Essential Low Block	→	✓	✓	✓	✓	✓	✓	✓	✓	✓	✓	✓
11. The Bond of Rectitude	→	→	→	→	✓	✓	✓	✓	✓	✓	✓	✓
12. The Open Spiral	→	→	→	→	→	✓	✓	✓	✓	✓	✓	✓
13. The Open Double Spiral	→	→	→	→	→	→	✓	✓	✓	✓	✓	✓
14. The Guard of the Novice	→	→	→	→	→	→	→	✓	✓	✓	✓	✓

PEDAGOGICAL CHART

	Week 1	2	3	4	5	6	7	8	9	10	11	12
Month:	1st Month				2nd Month				3rd Month			
INITIAL STEP TECHNIQUES												
15. The Way	→	✓	✓	Studied within the development of subsequent techniques.								
16. The Applied Way	→	→	✓	✓ Studied within the development of subsequent techniques.								
17. The Way and the Force of the Spiral	→	→	→	✓	✓	✓	✓	✓	✓	✓	✓	✓
INITIAL STEP TECHNIQUES												
18. The Way and the Force of the Double Spiral	→	→	→	→	→	→	→	✓	✓	✓	✓	✓
19. The Way and the Essential Low Block	→	→	→	→	✓	✓	✓	✓	✓	✓	✓	✓
20. The Way and the Bond of Rectitude	→	→	→	→	→	✓	✓	✓	✓	✓	✓	✓
21. The Way and the Open Spiral	→	→	→	→	→	→	✓	✓	✓	✓	✓	✓
22. The Way and the Open Double Spiral	→	→	→	→	→	→	→	✓	✓	✓	✓	✓
INITIAL FOOT TECHNIQUES												
23. The Whip Foot, Middle	→	→	→	✓	✓	✓	✓	✓	✓	✓	✓	✓
24. The Whip Foot, Low	→	→	→	→	→	✓	✓	✓	✓	✓	✓	✓
25. The Whip Foot, High	→	→	→	→	→	✓	✓	✓	✓	✓	✓	✓
*Breathing Technique	✓	✓	✓	✓	✓	✓	✓	✓	✓	✓	✓	✓
Part 3. Forms of Reaction												
26. The Efficiency of Simplicity	→	→	→	→	→	→	✓	✓	✓	✓	✓	✓
27. The Spark of Opposing Forces	→	→	→	→	→	→	→	→	✓	✓	✓	✓
28. The Force of Two	→	→	→	→	→	→	→	→	→	→	✓	✓

PEDAGOGICAL CHART

Week Number:	1	2	3	4	5	6	7	8	9	10	11	12
Month:		1st Month				2nd Month				3rd Month		
29. The Ineffable Double Spiral	→	→	→	→	→	→	→	✓	✓	✓	✓	✓
30. The Fish That Escapes	→	→	→	→	→	→	→	→	→	✓	✓	✓
31. The Force of a Direct Reaction	→	→	→	→	→	→	→	→	→	→	→	✓

MEDITATION AND CLOSING THE CLASS

	1	2	3	4	5	6	7	8	9	10	11	12
32. *Breathing Technique of the Inner Power	✓	✓	✓	✓	✓	✓	✓	✓	✓	✓	✓	✓
33. Closing the Circle	→	→	✓	✓	✓	✓	✓	✓	✓	✓	✓	✓

Approximate Length of Class: 20 min.   25 min.   30 min.   40 min.   45 min.

Chapter 2

Boabom Jass-U,
or The Art of
Osseous Awakening

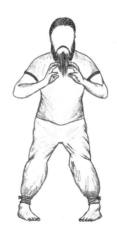

*Constancy has given shape to every form of life
that you know, even your own.
If you wish to trespass the frontiers of dreams,
you must know this last discipline.*

—*Alsam, from* Bamso, The Art of Dreams

First Part of the Class

ALL OF THE ARTS within our teaching have two essential stages. The readers of *Seamm-Jasani* will recall that the systems of movement within that book were divided into two great sections: The Art of Awakening and The Art of Eternal Youth, which is the technique itself.

In the case of Boabom, as I have said before, we follow a very similar scheme. Therefore we begin with the Boabom Jass-U, or the Art of Osseous Awakening, a system of necessary warm-ups and a way to begin the activation of your physical-psychical energy. This will let you develop the second part of the class (chapter 3) without a hitch. For ease of understanding, I have simplified this into three great cycles: I. Standing Movements; II. Movements on the Floor; and III. Ending, Closing Movements. Each cycle contains a stage of exercises, and all of these exercises are numbered from 1 to 20. The theory behind all of this is explained in the First Step, chapter 5 of the story.

Take into account that the process developed in this book is only a basic summary; however, as a complement to these exercises, you may alternate them with those shown in the Seamm-Jasani book, especially those related to cervical (neck) movements and sight. In this way you will have a better preparatory development, more complete and exact.

Welcome!!!

Cycle I. Standing Movements

1. Base Position

Before you begin, it is good to get an idea of something as simple as standing. Every time, within the movements, we speak of the Base Position, we will be referring to this form of standing, as shown in figures A and B.

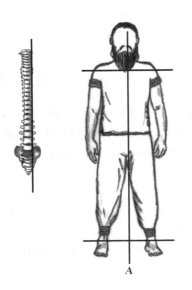

A

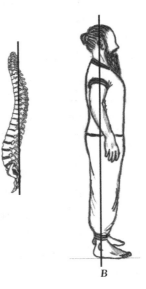

B

In general, keep the feet shoulder width apart, the legs straight, and the arms hanging naturally at the sides. From the lateral view, more or less, the ears, shoulder joint, lumbar area, and hip should be approximately in the same line. The head should be centered, and as the lateral figure shows, the back should show the natural curve of the spine, without any tension. This is the power of the arch in action.

Thus, from following these figures, you might learn something as forgotten as it is obvious: how to stand and keep yourself straight in a simple and comfortable way. It is essential that you have a strong base for the posterior exercises, for *their optimum development will depend on this*. All of them are related directly to this position. Besides, you will see that the physical energy released in this Art is centered in the spine and in its relation to the limbs. Also, having a bad physical position can bring pain and discomfort, the structure of the body being directed in the wrong way, causing an imbalance in the various loads and tensions that support the tissues. Most likely, any pains in your body are a warning that there is something wrong that must be fixed . . . and the time has come!

On the other hand, the way in which we stand can tell us much about our internal energy and how we project ourselves to the external world. Thus to begin the development of our Inner Power, we shall begin with something very simple: changing our exterior posture . . . before life! This position is immediately reflected in how we stand or sit. Let's use our bodies to reach our minds! So let us work on this simplest point.

You will also notice that the position we tend to adopt reflects the work that we do daily. Watch any person who uses computers fanatically and you will see an example of how not to handle your back. (Lately, I unfortunately must include myself among those who suffer these computer ailments, though I am working to balance this business.)

Finally, it is quite probable that some accident or congenital problem, especially in the back or legs, may prevent you from doing the Base Position perfectly. Just try to come as close as you can (without hurting yourself!), be patient and give your best effort, and that is enough! Personally, when I was a child I had an accident and broke my right clavicle, which never healed so well, so one shoulder is a bit lower than the other. Also, around the same age, doctors told me that my knees were a disaster and that I would have many problems! But all of this did not matter to me, and the best thing about problems is that they are an excellent incentive to improve! (Ah! Someday I will tell the cause of that accident.)

Common Mistakes in the Standing Position

Through the drawings below, you can see the most common mistakes in the Base Position. In drawing A, you can see, from a frontal

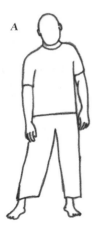
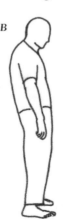
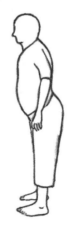

perspective, the figure out of balance toward the right, possibly as a consequence of what medically is known as scoliosis. In this drawing, the right foot extends to compensate for the imbalance in the body. Those who suffer from scoliosis should be especially careful in the execution of the posterior exercises. Drawing B shows the typical kyphotic position, the common ailment of the person who sits the whole day: the spinal column flattens and the hips move forward. When it loses its natural S curve, the spine loses strength and natural resistance, and obstructs the flow of energy, for Boabom depends on this S curve for a great part of its development and power. The last drawing, C, is the typical lordosic position, where the column's curve becomes exaggerated. This can produce pain and joint damage among the vertebrae.

2. Freeing the Energy: General Basic Movement, Relaxing

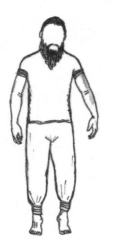

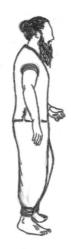

This movement is simple but essential in order to adapt, relax, and warm up. The Art of Boabom is a demanding path, and we need to be patient with our bodies as we learn to give them warmth bit by bit.

For that we do this movement (which we always call Relaxing) by walking in place with short but quick steps and shaking our arms as we move our legs. We will also use this between some of the movements in order to maintain the continuity of our movement.

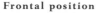

Frontal position   **Lateral position**

Our mind is now in a rush, wishing to be there right away, but we can give it only short steps. In this way, we begin to move heat, and therefore energy, to the limbs. When you feel that you are warmed up a bit, you are ready for the next step.

Symbolic Name: Freeing the Energy

Initial Position: Standing, Base Position

Breathing: At the beginning without breathing; once you are skilled in the breathing technique you can add the inhalation and exhalation, with two short movements: *nsss . . . nsss . . . haaa . . . haaa . . .* (See exercise 5.)

Affected Muscles: Structure and general muscles of the body/ general muscles and structure of the body

Duration: 30 seconds

Degree of Difficulty: 1 (from 1 to 5)

---

3. The Puppet's Advance: Hands at the Waist, Legs Straight to the Front

We are now ready for the true Osseous Awakening. We will begin by putting our hands at our waists, where they will stay as if they were glued there (see page 144, A). Loosen the legs.

We will immediately begin moving our legs straight and to the front, continuously one after the other (page 144, B, C), keeping them straight by not bending the knees at all, as a puppet with no knee joints whatsoever. Now the mind must demonstrate that it is in charge. The legs come back and forth, one after the other, faster and

BOABOM JASS-U,

OR THE ART OF

OSSEOUS

AWAKENING

. . .

143

A 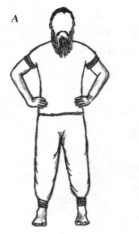 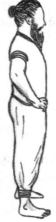 B 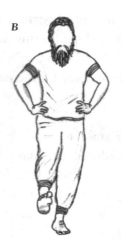 C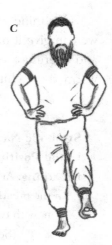

faster! The back and head we keep straight, trying to follow the line of the Base Position.

This type of movement strives to keep both feet from touching the floor at the same time. Instead, they take turns, out of phase with each other, one in front and one in back. After completing this exercise, we continue relaxing.

Symbolic Name: The Puppet's Advance

Initial Position: Standing, hands at the waist

Breathing: At the beginning, without breathing; once you are skilled in the breathing technique, you can add the inhalation and exhalation in two short movements, quick and constantly. (See exercise 5 and the note in number 9.)

Affected Muscles: iliopsoas, rectus femoris, tensor fasciae latae

Duration: Approximately 30 seconds

Degree of Difficulty: 5 (from 1 to 5)

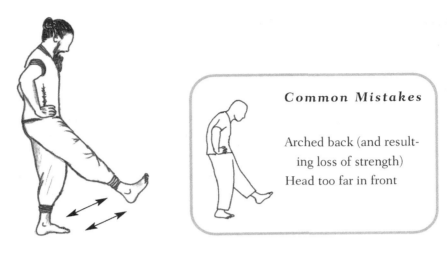

4. The Puppet's Retreat: Hands at the Waist, Legs Straight Back

After relaxing a while, we return to the same position as in the last movement, hands again glued to our waist. Now, however, our movement will be a bit more strange and complex: we will keep the legs as straight as possible (again, no knee joint!) and move them behind us, one after the other. Just as in the previous movement, we must do this exercise continuously and quickly, and if you can, do it even faster and more sharply.

This is a rather complex movement, which will measure the co-ordinative capacity of both legs. Normally, a beginning student will project one leg behind, following the drawing, but will then return it to the center (meaning that for a second both legs will be on the floor) before moving the other leg behind. An experienced student will no longer make this common mistake but will move one leg behind and while returning it will project the other immediately, so that

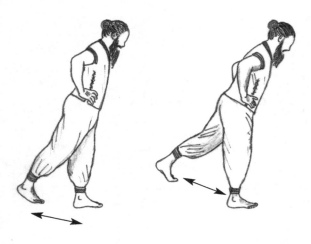

both legs will never be in the same place at the same time. The principle is the same as in Exercise 3.

Practice this exercise and you will come to understand and properly execute it. As I have said before, it is a complex movement, but when it is well executed, it produces a quick acceleration of the great bomb that is the heart. Afterward, we continue relaxing.

Symbolic Name: The Puppet's Retreat
Initial Position: Standing, hands at the waist
Breathing: At the beginning without breathing; once you are skilled in the breathing technique, you can add the inhalation and exhalation in two short movements, quick and constantly. (See exercise 5 as well as the note in number 9.)
Affected Muscles: Gluteus maximus, hamstrings
Duration: Approximately 30 seconds
Degree of Difficulty: 5 (from 1 to 5)

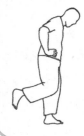

Common Mistakes
Neck arched, causing loss of strength
Back leg bent

5. Breathing Technique of the Inner Power

For the old student-readers of Seamm-Jasani, the explanation of this breathing will in many respects sound similar, for its base is very similar to the one we used in the Gentle Art. Despite this, and even though some aspects may sound repetitious, please read this section carefully, for you will see that there are both different details in the movement itself and in the application of this breathing technique. Remember that the Breathing Technique of the Great Circle of Seamm-Jasani has as its objectives the expansion of the lungs, which, combined with relaxation and stretching, produces the feeling of tranquility and rest.

On the other hand, the Breathing Technique of the Inner Power, which we will do now, strives to make the most of our breathing capacity, while strengthening our thorax and abdominal zone, producing a real defensive shell at the same time as we are capturing all the energy coming from this breathing, which produces a sensation of strength and vitality.

For those new student-readers who do not know Seamm-Jasani, do not worry, just follow the instructions carefully.

We will divide the explanation of the Breathing Technique of the Inner Power into three stages:

— The External Technique, or the physical movement itself
— The Internal Technique, or how you shall inhale, contain, exhale, and use the breathing tract
— The United Technique, or the technique in practice

The External Technique

We must begin in Base Position. Remember to keep your shoulders and spine straight.

(A) Hold your hands open and in front of you, slightly separated, palms facing the floor, at shoulder height.

(B), (C) Slowly bring your arms to your sides so that once they are there, both palms are now facing upward. The body does not move, standing straight.

(D) Now bring your hands in front of you, just in front of your sternum, more or less one fist distance from your chest, positioned as if you were holding a ball between them. At the same time bend your body at the hip but without bending your spine, which keeps its normal shape (changing only its angle to the floor); also bend your knees slightly and point your feet toward each other so that they face diagonally inward.

Look carefully at the drawings, for this is the most difficult part of the movement, as it coordinates the hands, arms, thorax, legs, and feet. Remember too that this part (D) is meant to be done all at once, not step by step.

(E) Remaining in this same position, turn your hands (and only your hands!), as if you wanted to see the underside of the imaginary ball you are holding in front of yourself.

(F), (G) Last, lower you hands slowly, turning your still open palms toward the floor as you project. As your hands come down and forward your body returns to its Base Position, where it began, meaning that the thorax comes back to vertical, the legs straighten and the feet, turning on the heels, finally returning to normal, parallel with one another.

The Internal Technique

Now I will describe the process of inhaling, containing, and exhaling.

Inhalation, Acquiring Strength

To inhale, you must first put your tongue against your palate (behind your top teeth). Then inhale naturally through your nose. You will feel a gentle pressure in your nostrils, and you will make a noise that I attempt to describe as "*nnnsss . . .*" though it is hard to describe this sound with letters and words. It sounds like a normal nasal inhalation, only more exaggerated, meaning that the person doing it should hear it clearly. As another example, I could say that the sound made is like that of a bellows or a balloon losing air (only that in our case, the balloon is being inflated!).

The idea is to maximize this inhalation. The air we obtain will be the foundation from which we will produce the Inner Power. If the inhalation is deficient or too short, your Inner Power will not have the elements necessary to achieve its maximum expression. The air too must be digested, acquiring heat, fluidity, and purity.

While inhaling, we use the thoracic cavity to its maximum, as well as the diaphragm, and therefore the stomach. This means that we are amplifying the thorax to its maximum simultaneously as we are lowering the diaphragm, and with this using all of our capacity, turning into a kind of balloon. Look carefully at the drawing. The arrows indicate the direction of both the air and the forces in motion.

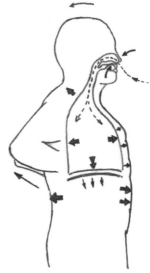

Containment, Feeding the Inner Power

Now we must contain all of the air. This is the climax in the action of what I have called the Inner Power, but remember that, as with every climax, its duration is ephemeral. Later I will explain how this process of containment, when combined with the external stage (the movements) can produce an incredible defense, making highly resistant a series of points that would normally be considered rather weak. Now, this is not about any circuses (which, unfortunately, the great masses adore), or walking around and telling a friend to hit you in the stomach with a stick, or leaning against a spear to prove your powers; let us leave those games to the ignorant and dedicate ourselves to the real Art as it was in its origin, in solitude and without exaggeration.

Exhalation, Extending the Inner Power

Now we will release the tongue, letting it drop from the palate, and exhale, but first we must round the lips (they will take the form of an O), and gently force the air passing through the throat, scratching it softly, making a sound something like "*hhhaaa....*" Though the lips are rounded, this sound is somewhere between an "Ah" and an "Oh."

As an example, the sound could be compared to exhaling through the mouth with a congested throat.

A natural pressure will be produced there, in the throat, but at the same time we will be working with the stomach, holding it in tension, flexed, through all of the exhalation. Do not make the mistake of loosening it immediately; work with the abdominal area to make it accompany the exhalation step by step. In the drawing on page 151, the small arrows indicate the flow of air and its pressure, while the large arrows indicate the work of the diaphragm and the muscles of the abdomen and thorax. These arrows are doubled because the muscles relax as they hold the tension and produce an opposing force.

Many people often practice certain breathing techniques in which they only blow the air, without making it work effectively. To identify and correct this mistake, we have to pay attention to how the air leaves us: if it leaves through the lips and mouth as if we were blowing through a straw, it is definitely wrong. You should not feel the air leaving by the lips but feel it escaping through the throat into the mouth, still keeping that tension in the stomach. Look at the arrows in the drawing, which also indicate the tension in the throat.

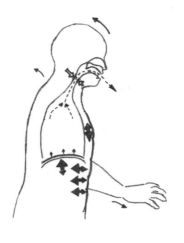

As we gently scratch the throat, we cleanse our breathing tract of any impurities that may be trapped there, at the same time our shield is strengthened.

It is said that in this stage we extend the inner force because, even though we are exhaling and we might think that we filled the balloon earlier, through the pressure of the lungs, thorax, and diaphragm, we will find that this is not actually so. On the contrary, we will continue to make the most of the energy that has been produced, allowing it to develop to its maximum.

This is an excellent exercise, but it must be done with precision and care. Its correct application will give you strength and will allow you to understand the real power of Osseous Boabom.

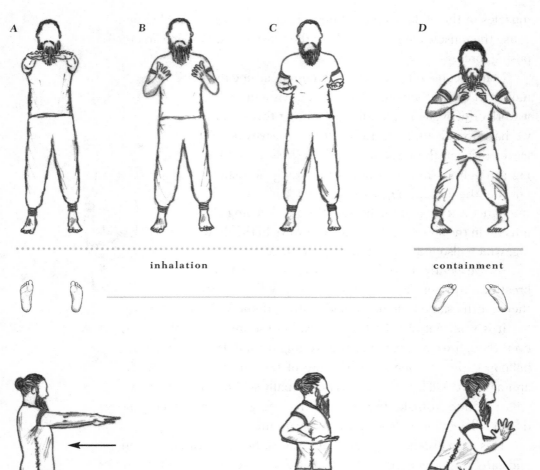

inhalation

containment

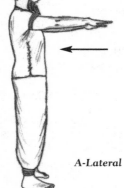

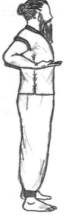

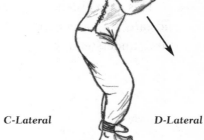

A-Lateral

C-Lateral

D-Lateral

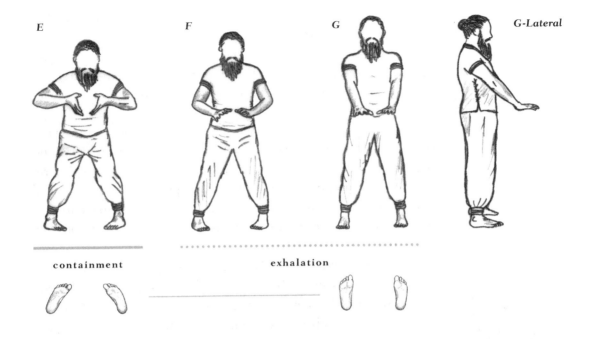

E   F   G   G-Lateral

containment   exhalation

The United Technique:
The Breathing of the Inner Power

The time has come to weave and link. Remember that the effectiveness of each movement of Boabom depends on the creation of the correct fabric of factors in its execution, whether they are technique, breathing, will, confidence, or energy. Now we are ready to develop the real Osseous Breathing technique, or the Breathing of the Inner Power.

In general, follow the figures above from the Complete Breathing Process. The detailed description follows:

(A) Beginning Position. Hands in front, tongue in your palate.

(B) Inhale (*nsss. . .*). Inhale slowly, as slowly as possible, and at the same time bring your hands to your sides.

(C) When you are finished inhaling, the thorax is fully extended, the diaphragm is pushed slightly down, and the stomach is extended a little. Once you are here, your hands at your sides, contain the air you have inhaled.

(D) Continue to contain the air, and immediately bring your hands in front of your sternum, as if you were grabbing a ball. Bend your body at the same time, but only at the hips—your spine remains straight. Bend the knees slightly and point your feet in toward each other. The abdominal area is flexed and hardened to its utmost, and both the legs and the arms gain firmness and some tension, too. This is the climax.

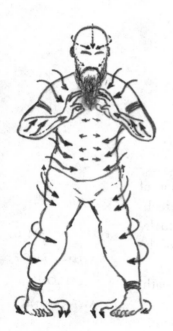

The Inner Power is born. In the figure at left, these Energy Lines symbolize the general tension produced through the entire body, and at the same time they indicate the direction in which this tension, or energy, moves: in the upper zone, the neck and the head, which lean forward; in the middle zone, the arms and hands, which face each other; in the tension of the abdominal muscles; and in the hips, which shift slightly to the back. They also show the legs, with the knees slightly bent, and the shins and feet, which turn toward each other while at the same time being tightly connected to the floor. All this at the urging of the mind, which must control the body as a whole and solidly center itself while commanding a group of parts that must work simultaneously together.

This whole process of containment and meditation (D) can last from five to eight seconds.

(E) Continue to contain as you rotate your hands upside down, looking at the bottom of your ball.

Energy Lines

(F) Begin exhaling *slowly* while lowering your arms bit by bit. As your hands descend, your body returns to its initial Base Position, with the hands in front, and the exhalation comes to a close.

(G) At the conclusion, a feeling of rest and general relaxation is produced as the exhalation finishes. In this moment the process is complete.

The breathing technique can be executed two or three times, and that is enough. Please do not worry if it is difficult or not perfect the first few times, for there are many factors that need to be done well in order for this technique to acquire its complete efficiency. One of these is the time to mature the technique.

Some Appreciations of the Breathing Technique

The breathing exercise itself is the most important segment in our Arts, in the gentle Seamm-Jasani as well as in the Osseous Boabom. You must learn it with patience, and persist in it until you understand it well and execute it even better! Remember that it is not only a way of breathing but also a way to meditate on your own strength and physical-psychical energy.

In the beginning, it is normal for your lung capacity not to satisfy you, but be patient and do not worry. The lungs are like a muscle: with time, if you exercise them they will develop and grow, and at the same time you can strengthen the muscles of the thorax, the abdomen, and even the diaphragm. When you have advanced in this technique, you will see that you can extend the time of your inhalation and exhalation without problems, but to get there you must go slowly, with patience and constancy.

If you are a smoker (of anything) do not worry, for this technique will help with your disease (sorry!). I mean your habit for tobacco (or

BOABOM JASS-U,

OR THE ART OF

OSSEOUS

AWAKENING

. . .

155

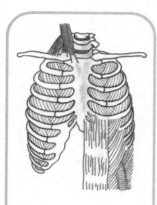

Muscles directly involved in the Breathing Technique: **External and internal intercostals, diaphragm, abdominal muscles, neck muscles, et al.**

who knows what else). I would like to use this opportunity to say that no kind of herb (legal or not) is good for your lungs, and therefore, for your brain, and for you. Do not believe those shamanic tales in which their supposed disciples need to smoke something so they can become enlightened, illuminated, or see some sort of light. In this case, the only light they will end up seeing is the light above them on the operating room table when they are having surgery for lung cancer, or perhaps on their brain! Please excuse the form in which I say this, but it is what I think! Anyway, the final decision will always be yours, and I can only say that our machine (body-mind) comes with all of the additives necessary to learn and discover great wonders on its own, and we need only learn to care for it, to value it and have a positive mind full of vitality, not full of smoke. Isn't there enough smoke in the city, anyway?

If you are a smoker, it is very likely that after a short time practicing this breathing technique, you might blow your nose and discover a very dirty tissue: these are the toxins that were stuck in your breathing tract and are being slowly detached, so don't be afraid. Take advantage of this efficient method to quit the bad habit of smoking once and for all. Forget the Exterior Smoke and live the Inner Power, and you will have surprises!

From the point of view of the Art as a form of defense, this breathing technique is vital for the execution of each movement. It will accompany all of the warm-up movements and every Boabom technique, so when, in the movements that follow, I mention inhaling or exhaling, I will be referring to the form described above, the placement of the tongue, the use of the throat, the shape of the lips, and the sound itself. Obviously, the external movements of arms and legs will change with each exercise.

With the breathing we can give speed to the movement, bring power, be more precise, focus the mind, and make each technique accurate while giving it a strength that is not usual. The idea is to use all this energy in an imaginative, inner way, to make it serve us as a way to give the maximum vitality to our body and, with it, to our mind. This form of breathing is also called Inner Power for it tends to produce a natural padding that cushions us against any strike we may receive, though the idea is neither to receive nor to give any such thing, only to use your imagination. Yet this cushion also strengthens our vital points and organs and strengthens the muscles of our stomach and thorax, thus producing the shield or natural defense I spoke of earlier. Also, the benefits of the breathing are always generous: it will help you to relieve a headache, overcome stress, even improve your digestion (for the diaphragm stimulates your whole digestive tract). But more than words, all of this requires constancy to see any results.

With practice, attention, and a positive mind, you will understand this technique well and finally come to truly discover what we have described as Inner Power.

Notes About the Application of Jass-U and the Osseous Art

There will be a difference in the application of the breathing technique in the Jass-U (this chapter) and the Osseous Art, or Boabom itself (the next step, chapter 3). When it is part of the Jass-U, the application will vary in each case, being lengthened or shortened depending on the particular movement; this is described

BOABOM JASS-U,
OR THE ART OF
OSSEOUS
AWAKENING

. . .

157

in detail in each particular case. However, in chapter 3, Boabom itself, you will find that the breathing technique must be strong, sharp, and quick; it should not be extended too long. In this stage, mainly with the hand movements (chapter 3, numbers 6 to 14), the breathing technique is like a spark that lasts only a second, joined at the same time with a strong and confident expression on your face, developing its natural power to the maximum. It might not happen immediately, but it must be your primary goal.

Common Mistakes

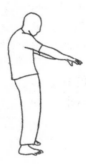 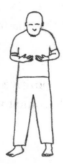 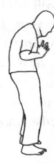

Arms too low
Hips tilted to the front
Concave spine

Hands in front
Shoulder in protraction
Feet unaligned
Lower use of thoracic
    capacity

Concave spine
Feet open or parallel
Poor development of
    energy

. . .

6. Harvesting: Lowering the Arm to the Side, Circular

This exercise can also be called Picking Rocks or Harvesting. Though it might sound a little childish, if we use our imaginations this can look as if we are picking up stones or something from the ground, and this will help us to understand its mechanics.

First, relax as you did before (A). In an instant, stop completely and bring the right arm straight behind you, with the palm opened in the same direction, fingers pointed upward, as if pushing something behind you (B). Now sweep the arm to the front (C) and inhale through your nose, as you have just learned. Watch your position, and do not rotate or turn yourself: the body remains straight, and then you slowly begin lowering your trunk by bending forward at the waist.

The trunk now moves forward, descending, and the hand begins to follow it, descending too, but in an arc, as if you wanted to reach something on the floor, as in the figures. The hand continues its trajectory toward the front, nearly but never touching the ground, while the body begins to stretch back (D). Begin exhaling now, until the trunk is straightened and the hand has naturally returned to your side, with the palm facing upward (E–G). In this instant, end the exhalation. (The total motion of the hand forms a semicircle, from back to front, and then is drawn back to the side once it is in front of you and parallel to the floor. Also, remember not to bend your knees.)

Continue relaxing now, back to figure A. Now stop again, and it's time to repeat the same, but on the left side.

The inhalation with this movement is strong, as is the exhalation. As you progress, try to push the exhalation to its maximum speed, to little by little, as we control it, make the movement faster and more precise.

A

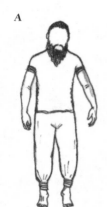

B

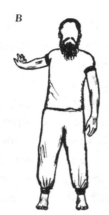

C

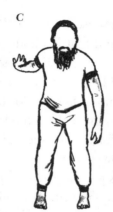

D

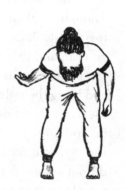

A-Lateral

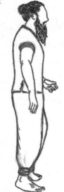

B-Lateral

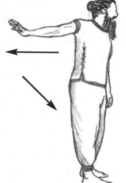

E-Lateral

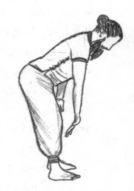

E

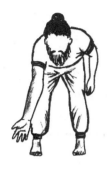

F

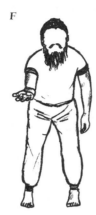

G

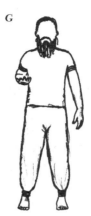

A

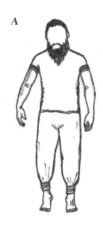

F-Lateral

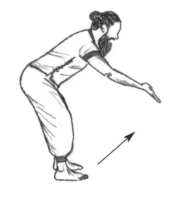

G-Lateral

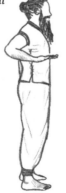

A-Lateral

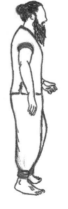

——————————————
inhale

· · · · · · · · · · · · ·
exhale

– – – – – – – –
**Releasing the
Energy**

BOABOM JASS-U,
OR THE ART OF
OSSEOUS
AWAKENING

· · ·

161

Remember that the work of the trunk must be centered more in the hip than in the lumbar area if you want to achieve the optimum results.

After the complete sequence, continue relaxing, ready for the next step.

Symbolic Name: Harvesting
Initial Position: Standing, relaxing
Breathing: Inhale when bringing the hand back and moving it in the descending circle (*nsss . . .*) and exhale (*haaa!*) when bringing the hand back to the side.
Affected Muscles: In the torso and legs: erector spinae, transverso-spinalis, rectus abdominus, stretching of the semitendinosus and semimembranosus. In the arms (and shoulders): rhomboids, triceps, biceps, latissimus dorsi, teres major, deltoid, pectoralis major
Duration: 10 times for each side, or 30 to 40 seconds
Degree of Difficulty: 4 (from 1 to 5)

Common Mistakes

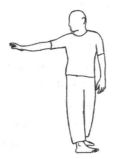

Turning the trunk when
bringing the arm back.
This error causes a lateral
turning of the body.
Feet unaligned

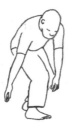

Lateral bending of the body,
which can impede the
work done by the spine
Crossing the opposite arm in
front of the body, bringing
a general imbalance

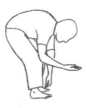

A complete arching of the spine, excessively forcing the lumbar area, as seen in
the drawing. Our objective is to bend at
the hip and, therefore, for the back to
keep its natural line as shown on pages
160–161.

BOABOM JASS-U,

OR THE ART OF

OSSEOUS

AWAKENING

. . .

163

7. Heel-Hand Game:
Relaxing to the Side, Heel-Hand

This is a very common exercise, though we will have our own variation.

Begin by relaxing normally. The movement itself is done by bringing the leg to one side, touching the heel to the hand as the drawing indicates, then alternating to the other side, but the movement must be done continuously, with speed and precision, so the feet never touch the ground at the same time: one foot is always in the air while the other serves for that instant as support, and then they switch roles. You must work with some speed for the movement to have grace, as well as its effect.

The other important aspect is that the leg is not only lifted to reach the hand (for that would imply a projection straight back) but also works with torsion to the side; this makes it a bit more complex and carries a certain risk, so take care. The ideal is to keep your

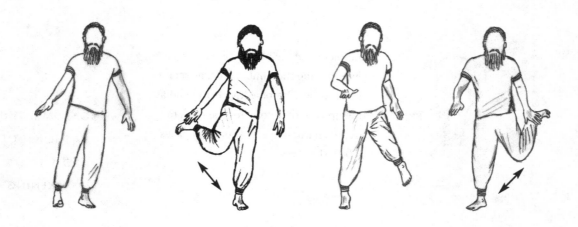

hands in the plane of your hips, but if you cannot reach that point, do not worry, be patient, do your best and with a little time you will see progress. If you have serious knee problems, definitely skip this exercise and move on to the next one.

Through the whole of this movement, keep the body's central axis in one line.

When you are finished, continue relaxing.

Symbolic Name: Heel-Hand Game
Initial Position: Standing, relaxing
Breathing: Inhaling and exhaling with two short breaths, quickly
and constantly (*nsss! nsss! haaa! haaa!*) (See the note in number 9.)
Affected Muscles: Semitendinosus, semimembranosus, adductors
of the hip, hamstrings, sartorius, gastrocnemius, popliteus, gra-
cilis, tibialis anterior
Duration: Approximately 30 seconds
Degree of Difficulty: 3 (from 1 to 5)

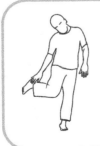

Common Mistakes

Turning the head to the side
Loss of the body's center
Knee too high

8. Touching the Earth: Crouching

Continue relaxing the arms and legs when you are beginning this movement (A).

All of a sudden, simply drop straight down (as if you were fainting or had lost feeling in your legs) into a crouch. When descending, without giving any resistance whatsoever, inhale, and at the same time try to touch the floor with your hands, as shown in drawings B and C. Try to keep your knees apart and your feet close together, just as in drawing C. When you stand up, exhale. Continue to relax normally, then drop again quickly.

In the beginning, a movement like this should not be too complex, but if your physical condition is just beginning to shape up you should go step by step, without rushing. So it is not necessary to touch the floor on your first try; allow yourself to drop only a bit: follow the example given in the alternative position, in which the hands do not reach the floor. With time you will be able to go lower.

Always keep in your mind that your spine must stay straight; do not lean forward.

After a moment with this exercise, continue to the next.

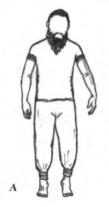

A

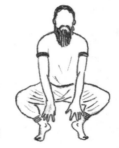

B

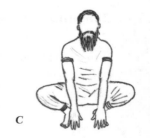

C

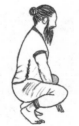

Symbolic Name: Touching the Earth

Initial Position: Standing, relaxing

Breathing: Inhaling when descending (*nsss!*) and exhale when rising (*haaa!*)

Affected Muscles: Quadriceps femoris, hamstrings, abductors and adductors of the hip, gastrocnemius

Duration: 12 movements, or approximately 30 seconds

Degree of Difficulty: 2 (from 1 to 5)

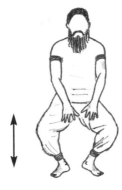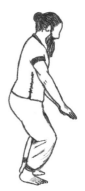

alternative
position

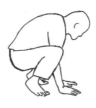

Common Mistakes

When descending, bending the spine from trying to touch the floor

Feet too far apart

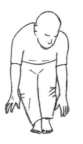

Descending only halfway

Feet too close together

Keeping the knees together, or holding them more to one side than the other

Lowering the back

BOABOM JASS·U,
OR THE ART OF
OSSEOUS
AWAKENING

· · ·

9. The Pincers: Fists Front to Front, Two Short Movements Back

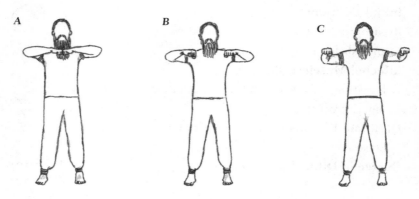

A   B   C

Now we stop ourselves completely and take a normal and comfortable standing position (Base Position). The idea is to work with the arms and shoulders in retraction. So bring your hands, in fists, in front of you, your arms making a rectangle in front of you, as in the drawings. Try to keep your arms and fists in one line at the height of your shoulders (A), neither higher nor lower. Keeping to this line is important: remember that the difference of Boabom lies in its details. Thus a good foundation makes a good building.

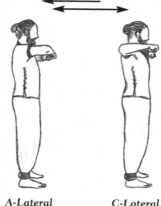

A-Lateral   C-Lateral

Now we pull our elbows back, keeping our arms at the same angle, as in figure B. This movement to the back should be done in two short movements, so we inhale twice, short and quick (*nsss! nsss!*). We now return immediately to the point where we began, exhaling only once (*haaa!*).

It is as though our arms formed a great pincer that opens and closes like a machine, with strength and speed.

After finishing this sequence, relax for a few seconds, including your arms, before continuing with the next movement.

NOTE: Please take into account that when I say "two short movements," I mean that, instead of making only one movement that comes straight back to its origin, the movement needs an insistence, or that is, it must be finished with an extra movement before returning. So once you have pulled your arms back, bring them back a second time before returning them to the front. When I speak of "two short movements" in relation to the breathing, you should inhale two short times (*nsss! nsss!*) before exhaling, which allows the air to be better used. The same thing may happen with the exhalation (*haaa! haaa!*), if required, depending on the exercise.

Symbolic Name: The Pincers
Initial Position: Standing, Base Position
Breathing: Inhaling and exhaling with two short movements to the back (*nsss! nsss!*) and exhaling with one movement to the front (*haaa!*)
Affected Muscles: Deltoid, rhomboids, biceps, pectoralis major
Duration: 16 movements, or approximately 30 seconds
Degree of Difficulty: 2 (from 1 to 5)

BOABOM JASS·U,
OR THE ART OF
OSSEOUS
AWAKENING
· · ·

10. The Fists That Hum:
Loosening the Wrists

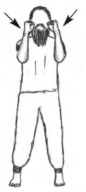
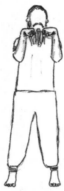

Prior position

Working position

This exercise is very simple. For those who have read *The Secret Art of Seamm-Jasani*, it will seem familiar. The objective here is to work with your wrists and relax your hands. It is especially recommended for those "sinners" who overuse their computers, abusing and damaging the tendons in their hands, elbows, or shoulders, or those with ruined nerves. Please forgive my sinner comment, for in my own embarrassment, I must include myself, though I always review my exercises (along with some other tricks), and in that way I release myself from the karma or hell of the sinners).

Now to the point. This exercise consists only of bringing the arms to the front and making fists, as shown in the Prior Position. Now bend the wrists, bringing your fists parallel to the ground, so they face each other.

Once in this position, rotate both wrists constantly, along the same plane, parallel to the floor, one in and the other out, then switching, without moving the rest of your body. Accompany this movement with the breathing, inhaling and exhaling. Imagine that your fists are humming, cutting the air in front of you (which they actually do, when this exercise is done well, after much practice).

To see in detail how to correctly form the fists, please see exercise 17. After a moment of

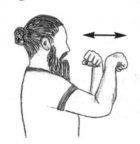
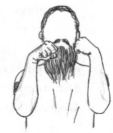

doing this movement, relax again, loosening your limbs, and then go on to the next movement.

Symbolic Name: Fists That Hum

Initial Position: Standing, Base Position

Breathing: Inhale and exhale continuously, one breath after the other (*nsss . . . haaa . . .*). The breathing does not have to be in time with the fists.

Affected Muscles: Supinators and pronators of the forearm, palmaris longus, flexor carpi ulnaris, flexor carpi radialis, flexors of the fingers

Duration: Approximately 30 seconds

Degree of Difficulty: 2 (from 1 to 5)

---

11. To Lift and Spill the Ewer: Standing Normally, Two Short Movements Down

This is another movement that will seem familiar to those who know a bit about Seamm-Jasani. It is a simple movement, yet complete and essential for warming up; this is why it should be, and is, in this book, although with some additional details in its current application.

First, take a basic position and hold your hands out in front of you, at shoulder height, with your arms straight (A). Now bring your hands back to your sides, turning them so that now the palms face up, inhaling with two short movements (*nsss! nsss!*) (B). Immediately lower your torso, bending at your hips and stretching both arms down

BOABOM JASS-U,

OR THE ART OF

OSSEOUS

AWAKENING

. . .

171

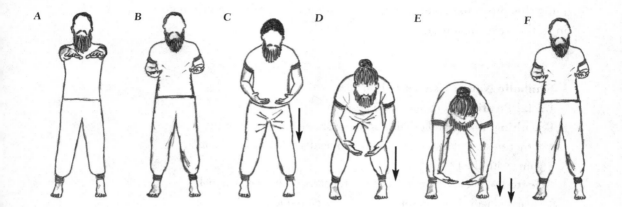

A   B   C   D   E   F

(C and D), palms facing up; when you reach down again make two short movements, exhaling (*haaa! haaa!*) (E).

The legs stay almost straight, though it is okay if you bend them just a little. Now come immediately again upward, inhaling twice again, with your hands at your sides (F), as if you had just picked up a pitcher with your hands.

Now continue, without stopping, going up and down with two short movements each time, continuously (sequence B-C-D-E-F).

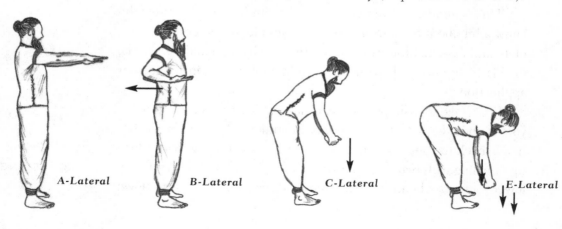

A-Lateral   *B-Lateral*   *C-Lateral*   *E-Lateral*

Imagine yourself a machine, full of strength, moving faster and faster each time, to your utmost maximum. When you reach this speed (but your real maximum speed!), slow down and then relax.

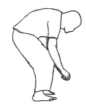

Common Mistakes

Bending the knees too much
Bending the back excessively
Incorrect placement of the hands
Feet too far apart from each other, or opened at an angle

This movement must be centered in the hips rather than in your lower back. Remember too that it is strong, and must be done carefully. Once you are finished, continue relaxing your arms and legs, preparing for the next movement.

Symbolic Name: To Lift and Spill the Ewer
Initial Position: Standing, Base Position
Breathing: With two short movements of your hands, at your sides, to the back (*nsss! nsss!*), exhaling with two short movements down (*haaa! haaa!*), in a quick and constant way, with the rhythm of the movement
Affected Muscles: In the arms: biceps, triceps, and brachialis. In the torso: erector spinae, transversospinalis, rectus abdominis. Also, stretching of the semitendinosus and semimembranosus
Duration: Approximately 30 seconds
Degree of Difficulty: 4 (from 1 to 5)

12. Swaying on the Mountain: Legs Apart, Two Short Movements to the Foot

In this movement, you must open your legs so that you resemble a mountain, as in figure A. Do it in a way that you demand a bit from yourself but at the same time at a reasonable measure, for this movement is not about "splitting yourself in two," as I fear some will try to do.

With your legs apart and both feet pointing straight ahead, take your left ankle with your left hand. Now with your right hand opened, palm facing up, try to reach the inside arch of your left foot, but in two short movements, inhaling twice (B and C). Now change immediately to the other leg, taking the ankle with the right hand and moving the left to the arch, in the same way as before, but exhaling now with two short movements (D and E). Immediately switch again to the left side. Repeat the movement, one side after the other, without hesitation. The change from one side to the other must be quick in order to keep the rhythm of the exercise.

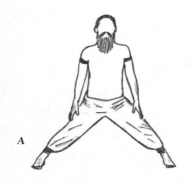

A

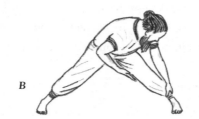

B

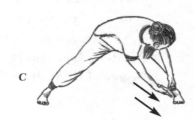

C

After you have finished the exercise, return to your normal position, relax your arms and legs, and then go on to the next exercise.

Symbolic Name: Swaying on the Mountain
Initial Position: Standing legs separated at a reasonable distance
Breathing: Inhaling with two short movements to one side (*nsss! nsss!*) and exhaling with two short movements to the other side (*haaa! haaa!*)
Affected Muscles: Internal and external obliques, pectoralis major, deltoid, abductors and adductors of the scapula
Duration: Approximately 30 seconds
Degree of Difficulty: 4 (from 1 to 5)

NOTE: Pay careful attention to how you grab the ankle, as well as the correct position of the hand, aiming it toward the arch of the foot.

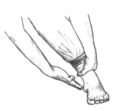

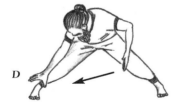

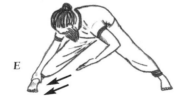

D   E

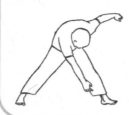
Cycle II. Movements on the Floor

13. Flight of the Butterfly: Sitting, Hands Interlaced, Butterfly

This cycle now covers those exercises realized seated and lying down on the floor.

Once you are seated, put the soles of your feet together and, with your knees bent as in the drawings, join your hands together under your feet and keep your back straight, as in Figure A.

Inhaling and exhaling normally, begin flapping your legs as a butterfly would its wings, each time a little faster, then faster, and faster, as if you wanted to fly (B and C)! This movement must be done with speed, and once you have experience with it, you will almost lift yourself from the floor! This exercise is very good for the thighs.

If you become very fast with this movement and someone takes a picture of you at the precise moment, it may seem as if you are levitating; as a matter of fact, this is one of the exercises that was used

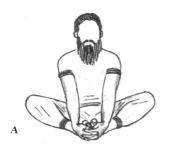
A

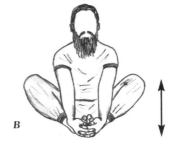
B

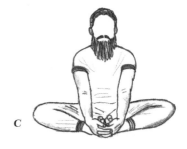
C

in Tibet to prepare for levitation, to make the body light. I cannot guarantee that you will fly, but I can tell you that if you are constant and careful, it will strengthen you, preparing you for Boabom.

Pay careful attention to drawing D, which shows how your hands should be interlaced in order to hold your feet.

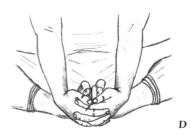
D

Symbolic Name: Flight of the Butterfly

Initial Position: Sitting, feet together at the soles, hands interlaced

Breathing: Inhaling and exhaling normally, one in and one out (*nsss . . . haaa . . .*)

Affected Muscles: Adductors and abductors of the hip, gluteus medius

Duration: Approximately 30 seconds

Degree of Difficulty: 3 (from 1 to 5)

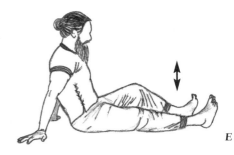
E

. . .

Once this exercise is finished, remain seated and stretch your legs to the front, relaxing them by lifting one, then the other, just a little, and preparing to continue (figure E).

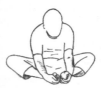

Common Mistakes

Bending the head too much to the front and thus bending the back to try to reach the feet more easily. As a result, not enough energy is generated in the thighs.

Bending the trunk to one side
Holding the feet incorrectly

All of these mistakes make the legs flap without strength.

14. The Embracing Bird:
Legs Straight to the Front,
Descending with Two Short Movements

Straighten your legs and begin with your hands on the floor at your sides, as in figure A. Now bring your trunk forward, bringing your hands to your calves and using them to help lower yourself a bit more. The impulse to the front is in two short movements, with two short inhalations (B). Now come back so that your trunk is straight up and down, and open your arms to their fullest extension, like a

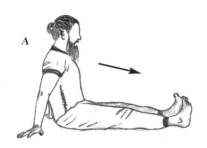 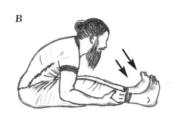 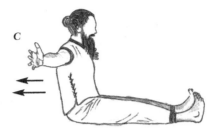

bird spreading its wings. This too is in two short extensions, and breathe with them. Remember that the movement and exhalation, just as with inhalation, must be synchronized (C).

Without hesitating or breaking the continuity of the exercise, return again to the front (B). Continue in this way, without stopping, until completing the sequence in the suggested time. Remember that there are always two short movements with the arms to the back, opening, and two with the trunk to the front.

Try to keep the natural curve of the back throughout this exercise, which means do not bend the back too much (see Common Mistakes). Try your best to follow figure B, and though your legs may bend a little, try to keep them as straight as possible.

B-Frontal

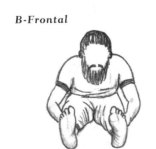

C-Frontal

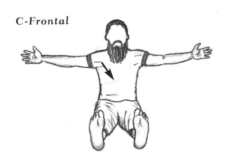

BOABOM JASS·U,

OR THE ART OF

OSSEOUS

AWAKENING

. . .

179

> **Symbolic Name:** The Embracing Bird
>
> **Initial Position:** Sitting, legs together and straight to the front
>
> **Breathing:** Inhaling with two short movements of the trunk, to the front (*nsss! nsss!*), and exhaling with two short movements of the arms, to the back (*haaa! haaa!*)
>
> **Affected Muscles:** Rectus abdominis, rhomboids, serratus anterior, latissimus dorsi, pectoralis major, deltoid, iliopsoas
>
> **Duration:** 12 times, or approximately 30 seconds
>
> **Degree of Difficulty:** 3 (from 1 to 5)

Common Mistakes

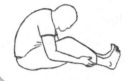

It is normal that when you are trying to go lower, the legs may bend or the lower back may curve. Both of these details are mistakes in the execution of the movement.

15. The Fish That Rises: On Your Back, Raising Yourself Abdominally, with Two Short Movements

Now lie completely flat on your back and make two fists, raising them over your stomach. Raise your head as in figure A and let your body follow, making two short attempts to sit up. Do not, however, sit up all the way; instead go only halfway, since the aim is to just lift

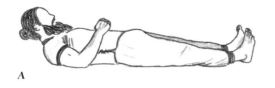

A

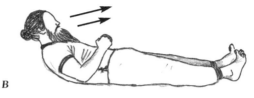

B

yourself off the floor a bit. You will immediately feel all the work in your stomach, which is where we want to center ourselves. When attempting to sit up, inhale twice, with two short movements, and when returning to the floor, exhale only once. It is important that you do not lay your head on the floor, instead always keeping it in the air for this movement.

Symbolic Name: The Fish That Rises
Initial Position: Lying on your back with your head up
Breathing: Inhale two times (*nsss! nsss!*) when going up (when making the effort) and exhaling once when coming back (*haaa!*).
Affected Muscles: Rectus abdominis, sternocleidomastoid, scalenes
Duration: 12 times or approximately 30 seconds
Degree of Difficulty: 3 (from 1 to 5)

Common Mistakes

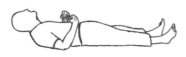

Not lifting the head before the exercise
Neglecting the correct position of the hands, and not making the fists well

Sitting Position

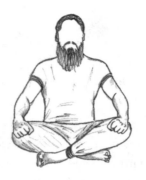 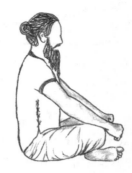

16. The Flower of the Inner Power: Sitting, Resting, Breathing Technique

Once you have completed the previous exercise, sit up with your legs crossed as in the above drawings, and prepare to execute the Boabom Breathing Technique. Following the instructions given for the hands in exercise 5, hold your hands in front of you, with your tongue on the roof of your mouth (A). Inhale with a long, deep breath while bringing your hands to your sides (B). Then bring your

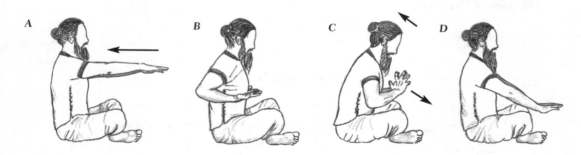

hands in front of your sternum as you contain the air, producing the internal force (C). Now turn your hands upside down, then exhale slowly, tensing your stomach muscles as you bring your hands forward and down (D). Remember to keep your back straight.

Symbolic Name: The Flower of the Inner Power
Initial Position: Sitting, legs crossed
Breathing: The complete breathing technique: long inhalation
   (*nnnsss* . . .), containment (. . .), and long exhalation (*hhhaaa* . . .)
Affected Muscles: Intercostal muscles, diaphragm, scalenes,
   sternocleidomastoid
Duration: Repeat the complete breathing technique twice.
Degree of Difficulty: 2 (from 1 to 5)

Do the breathing technique twice. Look carefully at the figures, for these clearly describe the correct position of the hands, as well as the appropriate position of the thorax.

Once you have done this twice, continue with the next exercises.

Common Mistakes

Among the most common mistakes are to lower the head too much and to bend the back. Another error is for the hands not to take the correct position, shown in figure C on page 182.

17. The Boabom Fist

Sitting down, lay your hands open on your knees with your palms facing upward, as in figure A. From this position, and with your gaze on your palms, close your hands, one step at a time, following the sequence indicated in the detailed drawings, until you come to make the fist, as in figure B.

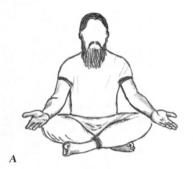

A

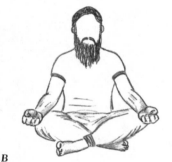

B

Here are the instructions step by step: begin with your hands open (P1); next, close the fingers as if you were looking at your nails, but without moving the thumb, and inhale (P2); third, hide your fingertips, tucking them in, and exhale (P3); and finally, close your thumb by bending it over your fingers (P4) and inhale, forming a strong, solid, and firm fist. Now open your hands again and exhale (P1 again). Then repeat the same sequence but with continuity and with no hesitation between repetitions.

This simple exercise will strengthen your forearms and fists enough to cultivate the Art of Osseous Boabom. You will learn, step by step, the strong points that a correct position of a fist brings.

On this subject, never listen to provincial traditions that say that, in order to strengthen your hands or limbs, you must break stones, bricks, wood, or who knows what else. Nor is there any need to put them in hot sand or in the fire. Leave that kind of circus side show to the movies; in the end, such tricks are nothing more than pointless bombast. If you wish to develop a true and necessary strength, simply practice this exercise. Besides, it is an excellent way to relax the hands from the tensions produced nowadays by our overuse of computers (which will only increase in the future!).

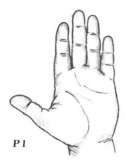

P 1

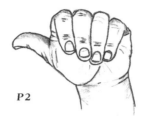

P 2

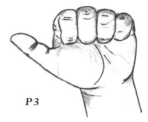

P 3

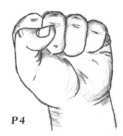

P 4

Symbolic Name: The Boabom Fist

Initial Position: Sitting with your legs crossed, fore-arms resting on your knees

Breathing: Inhale (P2), exhale (P3), inhale (P4), exhale (P1).

Affected Muscles: Lumbricals, flexors of the fingers, adductor and flexor of the thumb

Duration: 12 times, or approximately 30 seconds

Degree of Difficulty: 1 (from 1 to 5)

Common Mistakes

Not closing the fingertips correctly will keep the fist from reaching its necessary position, and this will prevent the thumb from closing as it should. This mistake is common for people with long fingernails.

In the drawing, the hand is closed well in general, but it has not reached the ideal angle demanded by this exercise.

18. The Boabom Palm

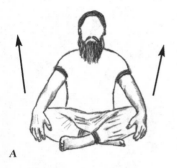

A

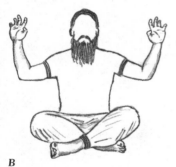

B

This hand position is a bit different, and is a highly effective way to strengthen and relax the hand, especially as a complement to the previous exercise. Simply lay your forearms on your knees, again with your hands open, but this time with your palms facing down as in figure A.

In one movement bring your hands up high, to your sides, with your arms bent as indicated in figure B. When doing this movement, inhale and hold your hands where they are for five to eight seconds. Then rest, returning your forearms to your knees, exhaling as you relax and loosen your hands (A).

The details of this position are as follows: first, all of your fingers are semibent, but in scale, meaning that the pinky is the most bent, the ring finger a little less, the middle finger even less so, and the index finger more or less even with the middle. Try to imitate, as best you can, the large drawing of the hand. Also, the thumb should always be placed firmly at the side of the hand (*not* in front of the palm) and bent; in this way, you are protecting it from any potential accidents in the quick movements you will be learning in Boabom.

The palm is straight—do not bend it, for that will take efficiency and energy away from this position. This shape of the palm is vital for a correct execution of these movements.

If you do this movement correctly, you will naturally feel a bit of tension in your hand, especially on the side. You will discover that this tension is one of the necessary factors in the different movements of the Osseous Art. Forming your hand in this way is like tun-

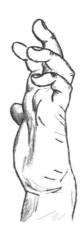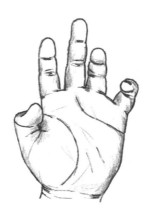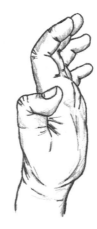

ing the strings on a concert guitar, or preparing a sailboat: if you know something of music or have ever sailed by the power of the wind on the open sea, you will understand me better. In this Art, each string of the great fabric of body-mind must be tuned to its perfect pitch.

Remember that each time I speak of the Boabom Palm, I will be referring to this movement and no other.

Symbolic Name: The Boabom Palm

Initial Position: Sitting with your legs crossed

Breathing: Inhale when forming the hand (*nsss . . .*) and exhale when relaxing (*haaa . . .*).

Affected Muscles: Extensors and flexors of the fingers, adductor and flexors of the thumb

Duration: 12 times, or approximately 30 seconds

Degree of Difficulty: 2 (from 1 to 5)

The drawings on page 187 show the correct position of the left hand when forming the Boabom Palm, as seen from both the front

The drawings on page 187

Common Mistakes

Here the palm has not reached its ideal straightness, and thus neither the side nor the fingers have attained the necessary tension.

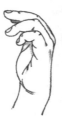

In this case, the thumb remains straight and the fingers too bent, so there is no tension in the palm, and the hand in general is too weak.

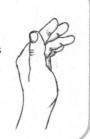

---

and the sides. You must pay careful attention, making sure that the palm remains straight and firm and that the fingers are flexed in the correct order.

Cycle III. Ending, Closing Movements

Now we come to the final cycle of the Jass-U. First relax (as in movement 2) for a moment after you stand up, in order to loosen the legs and let blood flow through them correctly, awakening them again after sitting.

19. The Balance: Leg Straight to the Back

Now stand in the Base Position and make fists with your hands in front of you, as indicated in figure A-frontal. Once in this position,

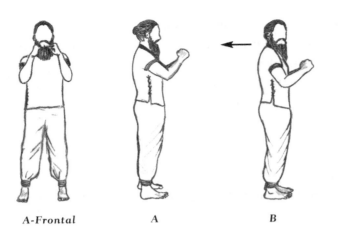

| A-Frontal | A | B | C |

look over your right shoulder (B). Now raise your right leg to the back, keeping it very straight (C), while at the same time lowering your body and continuing to look, out of the corner of your eye, at your ankle and heel. The leg remains as straight as possible, and you must keep your toes pointing to the floor, your foot straight up and down (D). When executing this movement, inhale when your leg goes back, and exhale when returning to the initial position.

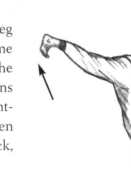

D

Pay careful attention that you do not bend your spine, either to the back or the front, but instead keep it straight and follow the drawings. This exercise resembles a balance, with one extreme represented by the foot and leg, which ascend with the movement; the other extreme is the trunk and head, which descend.

Finally, the fulcrum of this balance, its central axis, is your hips: this detail is important, for if this exercise is done poorly it can harm the back—so be careful! If you feel any pain whatsoever, simply skip this movement. Otherwise, be careful and precise and you will have no problem with this one.

Also, look closely at the lateral views, for they show clearly the complete sequence of the movement. Remember to always keep your arms firmly in front of you.

Once you have worked with the right side the indicated number of times, do the same with the left side.

Symbolic Name: The Balance

Initial Position: Standing in Base Position, making fists with your hands in front

Breathing: Inhale as you lift your leg (*nsss!*), and exhale as you lower it (*haaa!*).

Affected Muscles: Gluteus maximus, hamstrings, erector spinae

Duration: 12 times for each side, or about 45 seconds

Degree of Difficulty: 4 (from 1 to 5)

Common Mistakes

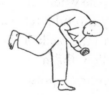

Excessive bending of the leg, and also of the back

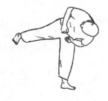

Turning the body, and therefore the foot, which ends up parallel to the floor

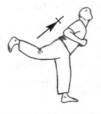

The worst of the mistakes: to arch the spine backward, causing excessive pressure

20. The Breathing That Closes the Circle

And now relax your arms and legs quickly, as you did in the beginning (see exercise 2). You can also drop your body, crouching, trying to reach the floor (see exercise 8). These are quick ways to energize the limbs and can serve as a final stretching.

After a short time stretching, relax, and close this cycle with two executions of the complete Boabom Breathing Technique of the Inner Power (exercise 5).

Congratulations!
You Have Completed the First Stage!

Now you are ready to begin the Boabom technique itself. Your body is well warmed up, your mind is alert, your senses have been stimulated, and the vital energy has been awakened! You are prepared for the second stage.

Chapter 3

BOABOM—THE TECHNIQUE OF THE OSSEOUS ART

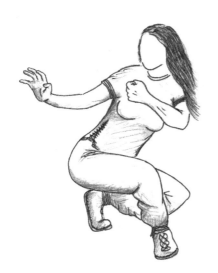

Work accurately with the bellows of the movement
For then air flows and blows with strength through the paths of the blood
That increase the flame which dances over the coals of the superior organ.
The mind extends and is tempered.

—*Nnuya, "The Smith," from* The Legend of the Mmulmmat

Second Part of the Class

IN THIS STAGE we will form Osseous Boabom, developing the different techniques as if they formed an alphabet, that is, first learning letter by letter, next uniting these letters to make syllables, and with time, depending on your perseverance, coming to be able to read continuously.

Take into account that the techniques developed herein form the most basic and simple beginnings of the great alphabet of our Art, yet do not take from this that they are superficial; each of them hides its secret, and though there are those who think they know everything, these first movements will teach them something new and ancient at the same time.

Generally, before starting these movements, it is a good idea to have warmed up thoroughly (by doing the Boabom Jass-U) in order to achieve the best results, for these movements are strong and require that the system in general be warm. If you have already read *The Secret Art of Seamm-Jasani*, you will be able to integrate it perfectly with this teaching. As for the application of the breathing, refer to chapter 2, movement 5.

I have divided this stage into six cycles, so that you may better understand.

— Stage I. Initial Positions: These cover the basic positions from which you will begin most of the movements.

— Stage II. Hand Techniques: Here you will see detailed the fundamental hand movements and their development.

— Stage III. Step Techniques and Applications: In this the basic steps are developed and combined with the hand techniques.

— Stage IV. Initial Foot Techniques: This will unfold the basic ways of moving the feet.

— Stage V. Study of the Forms of Reaction: Practical coordinations applied as an Art of Defense and projection of energy. This stage is developed in chapter 4.

— Stage VI. Meditation and Closing the Class: Here you will see a final stage, including meditation as part of the process of the class. With the previous, this is detailed in chapter 4.

Carefully follow the descriptions of the movements. Once you have mastered them, you will be able to execute them without need of this book; until then, each movement has drawings ordered alphabetically, frontally and laterally, which show progression of motion.

BOABOM—THE
TECHNIQUE OF
THE OSSEOUS
ART

. . .

195

Let the Pedagogical Chart (page 133) guide you. Go bit by bit, and in time you will discover the true speed of Boabom!

Through all of this stage remember that our greater goal is this: through the development of this teaching, you can discover your inner power, and for this, do not only consider these techniques as simple movements, but also use them as a way of focusing and projecting your psychical force. Through the combination of the physical and the imaginative you too will be able to discover the great potential that we all share; use that power, allow yourself to flourish in confidence, determination, and positive energy. Think positive thoughts, center your mind in each technique, and do not let yourself be bothered, distracted, or interrupted as you move through them. In this way you will be able to feel the complete benefit of this ancient Art.

Welcome to the Art of Defense and Meditation of One Thousand Ways!

Stage I. Initial Positions

Stage 1. Osseous Field: Position of Rest and Discipline

The base of the Boabom Art is discipline. In order to begin this Art, consider that this point is vital if we want any achievement or advance, whether physical or psychical. So within these initial movements we will begin with this one, which we call the Position of Rest and Discipline.

Stand with your feet together, your back straight, and your hands, in the Boabom Fist, held together in front of the area below your belly button. From this base will be born all the different movements and techniques, and at the same time you will emanate harmony, strength, and decision. This form is also used in the chambers of the teachings of our Art, for it represents a disposition of order and attention, the mind focused in Boabom.

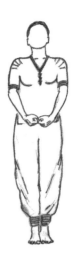

Symbolic Name: Osseous Field
Initial Position: Base Position
Breathing: Unspecified
Defense Application or Basic Objectives: Order, discipline, centering of the mind. At the same time, a basic defense of the genital area.

2. Normal Position of Balance: Normal Position with Hands at the Waist

Starting from the previous position, bring your hands up to your waist; this position will be used to execute many of the subsequent movements. The principal idea is to isolate the steps or movements of the legs, and in that way to center yourself in one facet, making your learning process simpler.

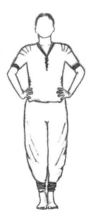

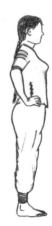

3. The Solid Fist and The Solid Palm: Normal Side Position—Fist or Palm

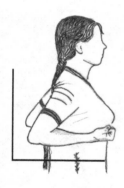

This third position will be another that you will use throughout the learning process. From the beginning you must be meticulous, as each stage has an objective that serves a necessary task in the evolution of this Art as a form of defense, as well as a way to increase our vitality and inner strength.

This position brings your fists to your sides. They are pulled back, the forearms are in line with the hands, and the back remains straight. In this way you are projecting the lateral zone of the thorax (the ribs), thus defending the back in a basic way while preparing to project in movements that use the Boabom Fist.

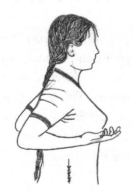

In the same idea we can apply the Boabom Palm, the open-hand position, with the palms facing upward; they too are in a straight line with the forearms.

4. The Fist That Is Born and The Palm That Is Born: Normal Side Position with Centered Palm

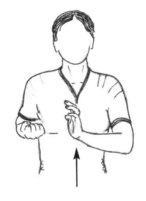

Based on the previous form, you can now learn another hand position that can be used simultaneously to begin individual movements and as a basic kind of guard.

Begin by pulling the right fist to your side, as in the previous movement, but this time open the left hand in the Boabom Palm and hold it in the center of your body, in front of your sternum. This same form can also be varied by using the Boabom Palm at the side as well as in the center. The type of position you use will depend on what kind of projection you are using it with.

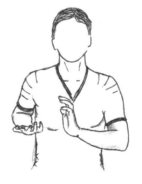

> **Symbolic Name:** The Fist That Is Born and The Palm That Is Born
> **Initial Position:** Osseous Field
> **Breathing:** Unspecified
> **Defense Application or Basic Objectives:** Protection of the lateral zone, front of the stomach and sternum, while preparing to strike

5. Universal Position

Within Boabom, there is a stage that we will translate as steps, which includes all the different positions in which you stand or move. In daily life, we tend to use three positions, or basic kinds of steps: standing still, walking, and running. In Boabom we have the same, only in a more technical way, with deep muscular work, while

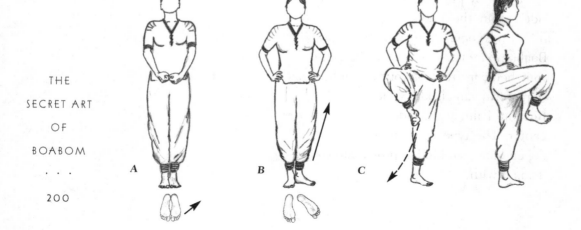

A   B   C

at the same time each of our steps has the objectives of defense and developing your energy.

The first of these three positions we will call Universal Position, or Arched Step.

For my student-readers familiar with *The Secret Art of Seamm-Jasani*, this will be a kind of review, but from a new perspective, with a different application from the one I detailed in my previous book. You must remember that Seamm-Jasani and Boabom are sibling teachings, each its own branch, showing its own perspective, of a higher science.

Now follow these instructions and drawings:

(A) Begin in Osseous Field; remember that the feet are together (as shown in the small drawing of the feet).
(B) Next, bring your hands to your waist in the Normal Position of Balance. Now turn your left foot 45 degrees, so it is open at a diagonal.
(C) Lift your right foot in front of your knee, with your toes flexed up (pulled back), inhaling (*nsss* . . .), pointing the sole of your foot at the wall.

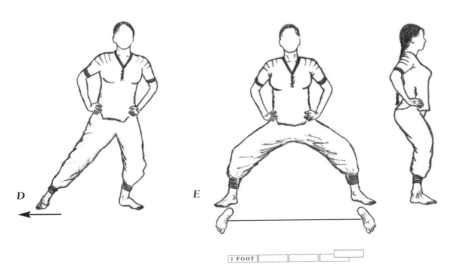

D

E

I FOOT

BOABOM—THE
TECHNIQUE OF
THE OSSEOUS
ART

. . .

201

(D) Now lower your foot immediately, exhaling (*haaa* . . .) as your foot moves down and to the right side. The foot follows a soft descent over a concave path, as if a landing airplane, until it gently touches the floor.

(E) In this, the final position, the legs form an arch, just as the drawings show. Your feet are approximately four and a half feet apart (feet as measured by your own feet since this length varies from student to student). Keep your back straight, perpendicular to the floor, following the natural shape of the spinal column. A good position will give you a strong, solid base. Bending the knees helps to protect them, as well as the feet.

(F) Now it is time to go back to the beginning. Keeping your hands on your waist, turn your right foot slightly inward and bring your leg back, inhaling (*nsss* . . .) in the exact inverse movement: your right leg takes off and comes up in front of the left knee by the same path as it descended.

(G) Finally, lower the foot as you exhale (*haaa* . . .), bringing your feet back together. Complete this movement by closing the left foot and returning your hands to exactly where you began: the Osseous Field.

Generally in our classes, this position is used mainly as an opening to the right side, but it can definitely be practiced to the other side as well.

This position is very common in many techniques of Eastern origin, but our way of applying it is as different as it is ancient. For Boabom, in its stage of defense, lifting the leg at the beginning is a way of defending your lower zone, but also, as the foot descends, its trajectory can be used as a very strong and effective projection. As I said before, this final position, the arch, is very safe and stable; to retain this, the feet should remain slightly open but not too much, for if they are turned too far out, we will lose our stability. The bent knee also ensures its firmness before any impact; it also creates a sort of shadow that makes any strike to the instep more difficult, defending these points that are delicate by their nature.

Besides, a good position provides the necessary tension for osseous and muscular work, which will be beneficial to your general health as well as, more specifically, to your thighs, gluteus, and all of your lower zone. For practice, you can repeat this movement three or four times and continue with the rest of the hand movements, all of which will be born from this position.

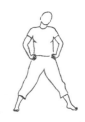

Common Mistakes

Not bending the knees enough (or bending them too much, which can produce an excessive load on the thighs)

Opening one foot more than the other, which causes an imbalanced position

Bending the head to one side, again causing a general loss of the desired balance

---

Symbolic Name: Universal Position, Arched Step

Initial Position: Osseous Field

Breathing: Inhale when lifting the foot (*nsss . . .*) and exhale as you step to the side (*haaa . . .*).

Duration: Normally we apply this movement two times between each technique that uses this position.

Defense Application or Basic Objectives: Balance and stability, defense of the knees and feet, form of projection

BOABOM—THE
TECHNIQUE OF
THE OSSEOUS
ART

. . .

203

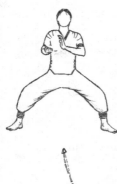

6. *The Force of the Spiral—Middle:*
Individual Projection, Middle

This movement has as its symbolic name The Force of the Spiral. As you come to know it you will understand the reason behind this name; analyze it with care. I have explained this movement in more detail, with many extra drawings, for this is a fundamental technique from which others, more complex, will be developed.

First, begin with the Universal Position, Arched Step, opening just as described in the previous movement. Once you are in a stable position, put your hands into technique number 4, The Fist That Is Born (A). The right hand makes the Boabom Fist at your side, while the left makes the Boabom Palm in front of your sternum: follow the drawings. Now you will apply the first movement of the fist in Boabom. It is a basic step toward understanding the secrets of this Art.

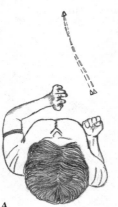

A

(A) Keep your back straight, the Universal Position firm and comfortable. Your shoulders should remain fixed throughout the movement, never moving forward or back. Your hands should be in The Fist That Is Born.

(B) Now, at the same time, move the right hand forward from your side, and bring your left hand back to your left side, forming a fist, all as you inhale (*nsss* . . .).

(C) Continue to project your right hand, turning it slowly as it ad-

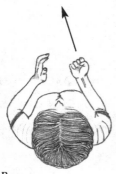

B

vances, while at the same time continuing to make a fist as you bring your left hand back.

(D) Finally, as your hand reaches its fullest extension, rotate it completely, finishing the spiral in the center line of the body. If you turn it too early, you can conduct the energy to your elbow instead of in front of you, which can damage your elbow. At the same time, the left hand has reached its normal position at your side, your left elbow pulled back as far as you can. Pay attention to this process.

(E) Now we follow the same sequence but in reverse: bring your right hand back as you extend your left forward, turning it in the same spiral, all as you exhale (*haaa . . .*). See drawings E-1 through E-5, lateral.

(F) Project the right arm again, this time sharply, with speed, and a short inhalation (*nsss!*). Contain the air for two seconds, then project the left fist in the same way, sharp and quick, with a short exhale (*haaa!*), and so on.

Execute this technique about twelve times on each side. After this, bring your hands to your waist and then your foot up and back, closing the Universal Position, Arched Step. Then rest in the Osseous Field.

Boabom uses a unique form, based on a quintuple force concentrated in the power of the arm and its projection, its spiral, the final rotation, the force generated by the other, returning arm, and the solidity of the Base Position. In general, a projection of this kind, in any of the common Eastern arts, would be straight; with no offense intended, that is only for beginners. The mountain is difficult, and only for the few, its jewels even more difficult to discover. Anyone who wishes to uncover the profound energy (and

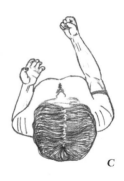

C

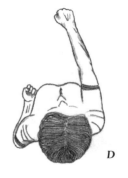

D

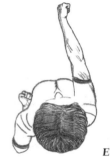

E

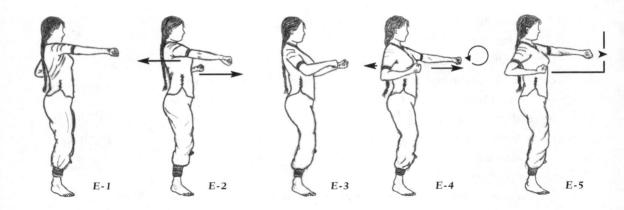

E-1   E-2   E-3   E-4   E-5

defense) that Boabom can produce will have to climb the difficult hillside and begin studying the incredible power hidden in its spirals!

In order to properly understand this movement, the student must pay attention to certain details and aspects related to the five elements I have called the quintuple force. Look carefully at the lines of force in the large drawing, as these will give you a more accurate idea of what the arm can generate.

In general, consider the following:

1. The projection of power works by a double effect: one part of its strength is directed to the front, while an equal strength is directed to the back, focused in the elbow.

2. All the power projected from the arm is in the major knuckles, those of the index and middle finger (what we call the Twin Mountains); the other knuckles are not used, for they have no support from behind, and in case of any impact they would be easily harmed. On the other side, the elbow sticking out behind you becomes a precise weapon that can defend in back, if that is necessary.

3. The fist must arrive at its goal at a medium height, approximately at the sternum, and centered in the middle line of the body, as shown in the top-view drawings. These axes should serve as a reference.

4. The fist must take a slightly curved shape, adapted so that all the energy of impact is centered in the Twin Mountains, which are in line with the structure of the arm: ulna, radius, and humerus. See the drawings at right, from the top.

5. The inhalation and exhalation in these movements is quick, with a sharp sound, bringing the same out of the technique itself: breathing and fist shall be as lightning!

6. Between inhalation and exhalation, that is, between the projection of one side and that of the other, make sure to *rest for a couple of seconds* (in this moment, your stomach remains tense, and after exhaling you will still contain some air, your lungs never totally empty). Acting in a quick and efficient way does not mean throwing one movement after the other, without order, striving for a continuous speed, which would only be a waste of time and energy.

7. The mind must be totally focused in this technique: isolate yourself from external thoughts, problems, worries, or ambitions. Live the movement. As you devote yourself to this technique more faithfully and technically, you will feel the Inner Power being born inside you; therefore you must center yourself in the movement, assimilate it, cultivate it, and follow the technique rigorously. If you do, you will discover that this movement is executed like lightning, a spark, and that the mind works in

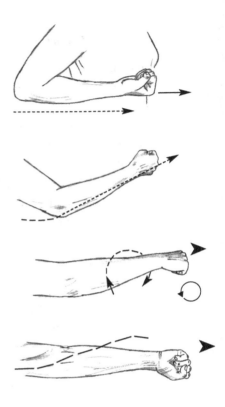

BOABOM—THE

TECHNIQUE OF

THE OSSEOUS

ART

. . .

207

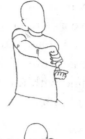

Common Mistakes

Lifting the shoulder or pulling it to the front, which distorts the movement

Bending the wrist, which loses the point of force localized in the large knuckles

Forming the fist poorly before beginning the movement, which causes the hand to finish in the wrong position

the same way, generating a great positive and expansive power. Think that the energy is born in the center of the mind and in a flash slides through the arm like lightning until it reaches the Twin Mountains. This way of channeling your energy can be used in all subsequent movements.

The effectiveness of this Art as a method of cultivating our energy and inner strength depends upon the precision and fidelity of our execution. Remember that this is the Art of One Thousand Ways but also of One Thousand Details. The old stories of this Art say that its loss and deformation by imitators through the centuries has generated much confusion; this has been because one student who was taught one thousand details did not notice four, and kept some others for himself, thus transmitting only nine hundred sixty, and his follower did not notice eight, and kept yet others for himself, and taught only nine hundred, and so on, successively, until later a new successor felt that what had been taught him was useless, as if you had a nice car with no engine. Nowadays, the heirs of these characters make big circuses and tournaments, break things with their heads, boast and carry flags of their nations, as if humans were born different, depending on their geographical circumstance, and nothing is left of the real teaching—the engine (and its spark!) were unfortunately lost a long time ago.

I take the time to remind you of this moral: that you must be meticulous and precise in your study and learning. Boabom is also the Art of the fine things, of the invisible. The one who understands it will go far . . . and will find that which is sought.

> **Symbolic Name:** The Force of the Spiral, Middle
> **Initial Position:** Universal Position, Arched Step
> **Breathing:** Inhale sharply when projecting the right hand (*nsss!*); exhale sharply when projecting the left hand (*haaa!*).
> **Duration:** 12 to 16 times each side
> **Defense Application or Basic Objectives:** Defense of the sides, projection to the front (with the Twin Mountains), mainly to the sternum. Use of elbow in back as a secondary defense

7. The Force of the Spiral—Low: Individual Projection, Low

Once you have understood the first way to execute The Force of the Spiral, you can quickly begin with the downward application, a variant on the previous. Anyway, look for details and follow the explanation carefully.

Low Application:

Begin in Osseous Field and execute the Universal Position, Arched Step two times. After the second, when you are standing in the Arched Position, follow these steps:

BOABOM—THE
TECHNIQUE OF
THE OSSEOUS
ART

. . .

209

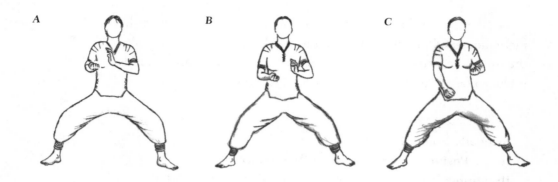

A   B   C

(A) The right hand makes the Boabom Fist at your side, while the left is open at your sternum (The Fist That Is Born).

(B) Now project the right hand forward and down, into the low zone, while bringing the open hand, the left, to your side, making a fist, inhaling (*nsss* . . .)

(C) Continue to project your right hand, rotating little by little as it advances, as your left hand continues back to your side. Try to follow the center line of your body, projecting all of your energy in the Twin Mountains.

(D) The final rotation is produced in the final instant, carrying all of the power. Observe the details: the wrist is slightly bent to take the precise form of the low movement, which is directed toward the floor.

(E) Next, follow the normal sequence of the previous movement: now bring your right fist to your side as you extend your left arm downward, exhaling (*haaa* . . .).

(F) Now project the right hand again, but quickly and sharply, with a short inhalation (*nsss!*), two seconds of containment, and then project the left in the same way, exhaling sharply (*haaa!*). Now continue in the same way, one hand after the other.

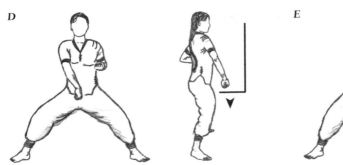
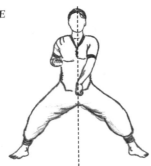

Execute this technique twelve times on each side. Then bring your hands to the Normal Position, Hands on Your Waist, bring your foot back and close the position. Rest in the Osseous Field.

In general, this is a short technique. You do not need to lower your shoulders in order to reach a point: simply work precisely with your arms and not with your shoulders.

Symbolic Name: The Force of the Spiral, Low
Initial Position: Universal Position, Arched Step
Breathing: Inhale sharply when projecting the right hand (*nsss!*); exhale sharply when projecting the left hand (*haaa!*).
Duration: 12 to 16 times each side
Defense Application or Basic Objectives: Defense of the sides, projection to the front (again with the Twin Mountains). The point of impact for this movement is the other person's Low Zone.

8. The Force of the Spiral—High: Individual Projection, High

Begin with the same initial process as described in the previous two movements, and get ready for another projection, this time high. Follow these steps:

(A) The right hand in a fist at your side, the left open in front of the sternum (The Fist That Is Born).

(B) Now, with both hands moving at the same time, project the hand in the fist forward, but this time toward the upper zone, while pulling the open hand back to the side as it turns into a fist. Inhale (*nsss* . . .).

(C) Continue to project the right hand forward and up until the movement finishes; remember to rotate your hand at the very end. The wrist should be bent slightly downward, for in this manner the Twin Mountains, and no other zone of the hand, can come exactly and simultaneously to the point of impact.

(D) Now follow the normal sequence of the movement, bringing your right fist to your side and projecting your left fist upward, exhaling (*haaa* . . .).

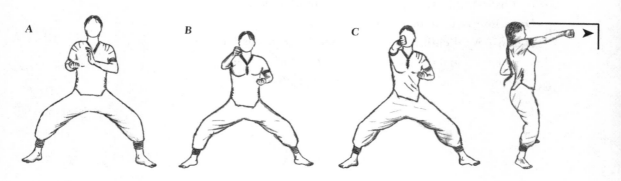

(E) Project the right hand again, but now quickly, inhaling sharply (*nsss!*), contain for two seconds, then project the left in the same way, exhaling (*haaa!*), and so on, successively.

Execute this technique 12 or so times on each side. Then bring your hands to your waist, Normal Position, and bring your foot back to close the open position. Rest in Osseous Field.

Symbolic Name: The Force of the Spiral, High
Initial Position: Universal Position, Arched Step
Breathing: Inhale sharply when projecting the right hand (*nsss!*); exhale sharply when projecting the left hand (*haaa!*).
Duration: 12 to 16 times on each side
Defense Application or Basic Objectives: Defense of the sides, projection to the front (with the Twin Mountains). This projection is aimed at the face.

Common Mistakes

Lifting the shoulder, which deforms the application

Flexing the thorax, either to the front or to the back, as in the drawing. Both these errors prevent you from establishing the requisite base for execution of the technique.

The retracted arm in the wrong position, or the wrist bent in that position, as shown in the drawing. This will prevent a properly formed projection.

BOABOM—THE

TECHNIQUE OF

THE OSSEOUS

ART

. . .

213

9. The Force of the Double Spiral:
Double Frontal Projection

Begin again in Osseous Field. Bring your hands to your waist and execute the Universal Position, Arched Step, two times. Once you are in this position, make sure that your back is straight and that the arch formed by your legs remains in a firm position.

Follow the development of the drawings along with these instructions:

(A) Normal Position, fists at your sides: The Fist That Is Born.
(B) Now, as you inhale (*nsss* . . .), project both hands symmetrically forward, following the drawings and using the same turning motion you already know from The Force of the Spiral.
(C) Bringing both fists directly in front of you, in the last instant (just as in the previous movements) twist them completely, projecting all of your force into the Twin Mountains, your primary knuckles. Remember to keep your shoulders in one line, not twisting them at all.
(D) After two seconds spent containing, pull your arms and fists back as you exhale (*haaa* . . .), completing this movement with both elbows pointing behind you, just as you began.

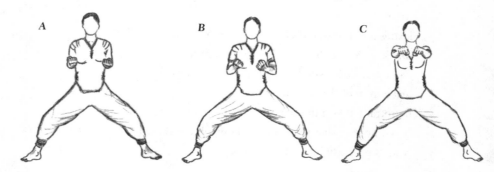

A   B   C

(E) Now you can project again, this time with precision and speed. Be sharp and powerful in your breathing technique, and remember that between each execution, front and back, there must be a short pause.

Once you have finished the full cycle of this movement, close your leg position and return to the beginning, in Osseous Field.

This is a very strong and complete technique. From the defense perspective, this movement can be used to stop a much larger, heavier, or stronger opponent. In order to accomplish this, the movement must be sharp, fast, and must precisely form the spiral effect, achieving contact simultaneously with both fists. Thus there will be four points of contact emanating all of the power: the Twin Mountains of both hands. Well-formed, this projection has no opponents. I write of this not with a warriorlike desire: it is not worth using the energy developed by Boabom for destruction when we can use all of that energy to develop what is within us; after all, there are already too many people busy creating wars and conflicts.

Common Mistakes

The double movement should be more simple to execute; nevertheless, if the previous movements have not been well learned, it is likely that you will repeat the same mistakes. In the drawing you can see how the shoulders can tend to rise, which is probably the most common mistake.

Other mistakes are to bend the arms toward the inside and to lower the head.

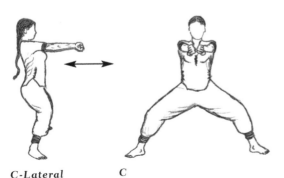

C-Lateral   C

BOABOM—THE

TECHNIQUE OF

THE OSSEOUS

ART

. . .

215

Remember that the perfect defense is the one never used.

> **Symbolic Name:** The Force of the Double Spiral
> **Initial Position:** Universal Position, Arched Step
> **Breathing:** Inhale sharply when projecting (*nsss!*); exhale sharply when pulling back (*haaa!*).
> **Duration:** 16 times
> **Defense Application or Basic Objectives:** Defense of the sides, forward projection to the thorax. Use of both elbows as a secondary, posterior defense.

10. Essential Low Block: Low Block

Begin again in Osseous Field, then put your hands on your waist and repeat the Universal Position two times. In this position, you are ready to learn a basic form of block. Follow these steps, using the drawings and descriptions:

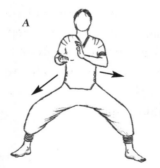
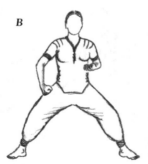
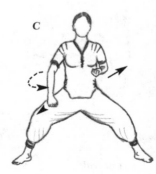

(A) Universal Position, firm and comfortable, your hands in The Fist That Is Born: right hand in the Boabom Fist at your side, your left hand open in front of your sternum.

(B) Project your right hand to the side, lowering it in a flattened arc, nearly a straight line, as you bring your left hand back to your side as it makes a fist (as in the previous movements). Inhale with this (*nsss . . .*).

(C) Continue to project your right hand downward, following the same line. In nearly the last moment, rotate the inside of your arm to the outside.

(D) This projection ends with this short rotation, and the point of impact is *only the side of the fist* (see detail). Your arm should not be totally straight but should remain in a slight curve, like an arch or a parenthesis. As all of this has been happening, your left arm has been pulled totally back, and its hand made into a fist. Remember that both projection and retraction should occur at the same time and that the shoulders have kept their line (D-lateral).

Now continue with the normal sequence: pull your right fist back to your side as you project your left fist down in the same movement, keeping the curved form and outside twist of this movement. Exhale (*haaa . . .*).

You can give continuity and speed to this technique. Inhale again with the right (*nsss!*) and exhale with the left (*haaa!*), using normal containment in between. Execute this technique twelve times

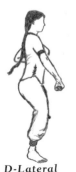

D-Lateral

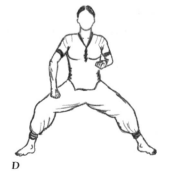

D

on each side. Afterward, return your hands to your waist, bring your foot back, and close to Osseous Field.

The objective of this technique is the use of the fist and the outside of the forearm as a basic block. The arm takes the curve I have described in order to protect your elbow, and the side of the fist serves to open a lateral-low zone, mainly to protect the area around the thigh. Look carefully at the drawings; the point of impact is the side of the fist, which is actually firm by nature (the zone of the pisiform bone). As every technique in Boabom, this has multiple objectives, as the same movement can also be used as a strike to the genital zone.

More important is that, at the same time, each link in the chain of this Art elevates your physical and energetic development, and remember that defense, in this case, is only for our imaginations.

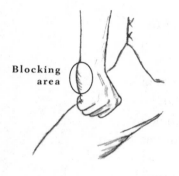

Blocking area

Symbolic Name: Essential Low Block

Initial Position: Universal Position, Arched Step—The Fist That Is Born

Breathing: Inhale sharply when projecting with the right hand (*nsss!*); exhale sharply with the left (*haaa!*).

Duration: 12 to 16 times on each side

Defense Application or Basic Objectives: Defense of the thighs or low lateral zone; use of the exterior of the hand as a strike to the genital zone

---

> **Common Mistakes**
>
> Bending the wrist excessively.
>
> Straightening the arm, which can cause the energy to move to the elbow instead of the side of the fist.
>
> Bending the torso to the front or pulling the shoulders out of the line they must keep to stay balanced.

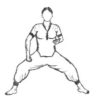

11. The Bond of Rectitude: Crossed High Projection and Block

After the normal repetition of the Universal Position twice between each movement, we move now to another application. This movement will be much more forceful and a bit more complex. Follow the explanation and drawings step by step.

(A) Both hands are at your sides in The Solid Fist. Project the hands symmetrically upward and in front as you inhale (*nsss . . .*).

(B) Continue to move your arms in their upward trajectory, the right hand now slightly above the left.

(C) In one quick movement, cross the right fist over the left at the apex of their projection, twisting them both one quarter of a turn so they are back to back, facing straight up and down. Your arms should be completely straight, your wrists bent slightly downward in order to allow the Twin Mountains, the two main knuckles, full exposure, forming a mass of upward projected power. (See the lateral drawings

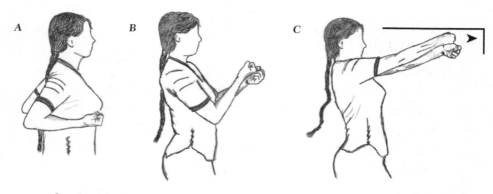

A   B   C

for the precise orientation of the hands in relation to each other and the rest of your body.)

After containing for three seconds, pull both fists back with the same power with which they were projected, and exhale at the same time (*haaa . . .*). Now both arms have returned to The Solid Fist (A). As you have projected your elbows back, you have also created a powerful field of defense behind you.

Continue with this technique, inhaling as you project upward (*nsss!*), containing for three seconds, and exhaling as you come back, with energy (*haaa!*). Execute this technique sixteen times, then place your hands on your waist and return to Osseous Field.

This particular projection, as every movement applied doubly, develops a great force and power. The difficulty in this movement is that both arms and fists work in synchronous motion, yet at the same time are crossed: they must arrive simultaneously in their final position and in the same way, always with the right over the left. In this way

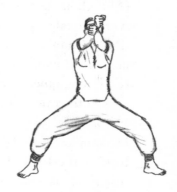

C-Frontal

you have formed two fists into one, which act as a block for high descending strikes. This form of block also acts as a strike, as it can project an incredible force to the high zone.

Symbolic Name: The Bond of Rectitude
Initial Position: Universal Position, Arched Step
Breathing: Inhale sharply when projecting (*nsss!*); exhale sharply when pulling back (*haaa!*).
Duration: 16 times
Defense Application or Basic Objectives: Defense of the high zone against descending or direct projection; projection to the face of the opponent using both fists simultaneously

Common Mistakes

Lack of elasticity or firmness in your arms can make you not straighten them as you should. This prevents the main knuckles from forming the straight line with the knuckles that is necessary for a solid movement.
Raising the shoulders is another common mistake.

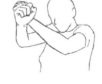

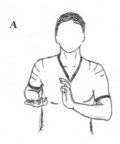

A

12. The Open Spiral: Individual Circular Projection of the Palm

Having executed the Universal Position again two times, you will now learn a new movement based on the open hand position and the use of the Boabom Palm as an element of defense.

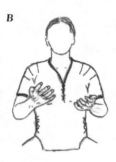

B

(A) Universal Position, firm and comfortable, your hands now in The Palm That Is Born: your right hand open at your side, your left in front of your sternum.

(B) Begin by projecting your right hand in front of you, turning it in a semicircle, as you pull the left palm back to the side. Inhale (*nsss . . .*).

(C) Continue projecting your right hand toward the middle as the palm slowly prevails to the front.

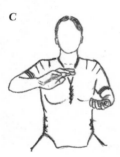

C

(D) This movement has reached its fullest extension with a slight curve remaining in the arm, and a final twist of the palm so that it faces directly to the front, as if placed flat against a wall in front of you. The exact point of projection is the bottom part of the palm, where it becomes the wrist, which has a great strength behind it. At the same time, the left hand has come to your side, keeping the hand open and projecting your elbow to the back.

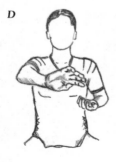

D

(E) Continuing in the normal sequence, now pull your right palm to your side as you project your left again with your arm arched and palm turned forward as you exhale (*haaa . . .*).

Continue, with energy now, and inhale with your right hand (*nsss!*), contain for a moment, and exhale with your left (*haaa!*).

Repeat this movement twelve or so times on each side; after you are finished, return your hands to your waist and close, returning your arms and legs to Osseous Field.

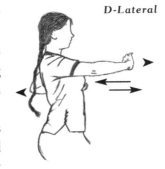

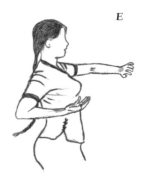

Now you must delve into this first application of the open hand or Boabom Palm. Remember that the power is projected through the arm into the palm but not to the fingers, since they are protected by being bent and are not applied in the contact of the movement. The arm remains slightly bent in order to allow us a more effective use of the palm and also to protect the elbow.

This movement can be directed toward the sternum: it is delicate yet dangerous. Work with precision and you will discover the true essence of the open spiral.

Symbolic Name: The Open Spiral
Initial Position: Universal Position, Arched Step
Breathing: Inhale sharply when projecting the right hand (*nsss!*); exhale sharply when projecting the left (*haaa!*).
Duration: 12 times on each side
Defense Application or Basic Objectives: Direct projection to the sternum, mouth, or stomach

BOABOM—THE
TECHNIQUE OF
THE OSSEOUS
ART

· · ·

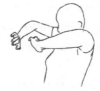
13. The Open Double Spiral:
Double Circular Projection of the Palm

After twice executing the Universal Position, you will learn the
following movement, which should not be too complicated since it
is based on the previous one.

(A) Initial position, hands open at both sides in The Solid Palm.
(B) Inhale (*nsss* . . .) while projecting both hands to the front, open,
without losing the shape of the Boabom Palm. Remember to keep
both hands symmetrical as they move forward.
(C) Twist both hands as they arrive together in front of you, projecting all the power of this movement into the palms. Keep both arms
slightly curved at the elbows, the fingertips of both hands almost
touching each other. Pay attention and keep your thumb closed and
firm and your back straight.
(D) After a moment containing, bring both arms back, pulling them
with force to the sides of your body as you exhale (*haaa* . . .). Your

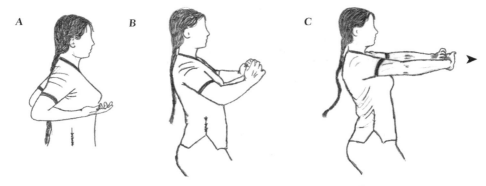

A   B   C

left and right hands arrive back at the same time, just as in figure A. Now all of the power has moved to the elbows, as has happened in all techniques of this kind.

Project again to the front, with a short, penetrating inhalation (*nsss!*); after a moment, pull your elbows back with force, exhaling (*haaa!*). Repeat this movement 16 times. Once you have finished this cycle, bring your hands to your waist and return to Osseous Field.

Just as in the previous technique, you continue to work here with the open palm but now doubly, in a movement that is very effective if you need to move a lot of energy in a short distance. The palm is naturally strong enough, and the double position you are now using produces even more strength, joined as it is to this short, semicircular movement. Its effect, especially when united with a step, can be immense (see technique 29, chapter 4).

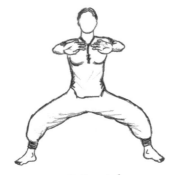

C-Frontal

14. The Guard of the Novice: Medium Block

After twice reviewing the Universal Position, get ready to learn a new technique, this one involving a basic block that protects the middle zone. The development of this movement follows:

(A) In Universal Position, hold both fists at your sides, in The Solid Fist.

(B) Inhaling (*nsss . . .*), the right hand ascends directly upward as the left hand ascends diagonally to the opposite side.

(C) Both hands meet, left crossed behind the right, forming the first part of the block.

(D) As you exhale (*haaa . . .*), raise both fists as you bring them to the front, left over right, descending along a diagonal movement both down and to the front. The left hand remains a bit in front of the right, where it will finish.

(E) Finally, both fists rest in front of you, both of your arms bent, left in front of the right just as in the drawing. We have now produced a

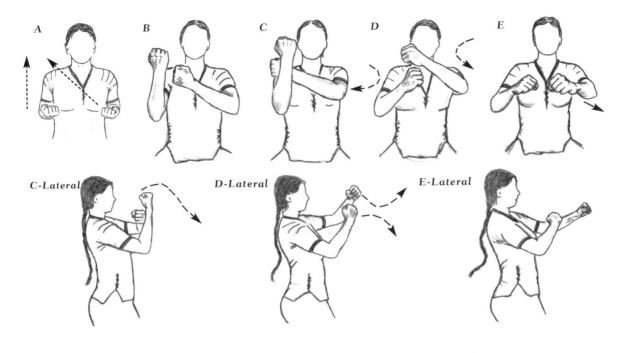

A B C D E

C-Lateral D-Lateral E-Lateral

double defense, using this as its second part, with the left hand blocking in front. The main zone of impact will be the side of each hand (the area of the pisiform bone).

(F) Now we will do the same on the opposite side, so inhale (*nsss . . .*) as you raise your left hand vertically and cross your right behind it, in a mirror of the same position as before.

(G) Exhale immediately (*haaa . . .*), your hands following the same trajectory of projection, but this time with the right leading and finishing in front. After two seconds you can execute the complete movement, continuously, to one side and the next, breathing in this same way but with energy (*nsss! haaa!*). Repeat it twelve times on each side. After you are finished, bring your hands to your waist and close to Osseous Field.

BOABOM—THE
TECHNIQUE OF
THE OSSEOUS
ART

. . .

227

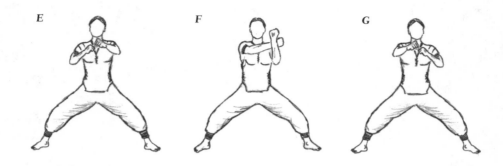

E   F   G

Within Boabom, we identify this kind of block as a composite block, as it combines many minor forms in order to achieve a complete block that acts as a whole. You can clearly distinguish the first part of the block (C), in which the arms and fists defend the upper lateral area; then, when the movement is projected to the front, another defense is produced, this time covering all of the middle zone, on both sides, with one hand in front and the other acting as a secondary defense. This technique can also be used as a basic guard, a solid and very efficient beginning form of defense.

Symbolic Name: The Guard of the Novice
Initial Position: Universal Position, Arched Step
Breathing: Inhale when crossing to the side (*nsss!*); exhale when projecting to the front (*haaa!*).
Duration: 12 times on each side
Defense Application or Basic Objectives: Block for medium strikes, covering the high lateral zone. General basic defense.

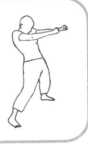

Common Mistakes

Overstretching the arms, as well as bending them too much
The general position of the body must be correct, including the
head, trunk, and legs. Otherwise, as in the drawing, the movement
loses its essential meaning.

Stage III. Step Techniques and Applications

15. The Way: Basic Step

This will be our second position related to movement of the entire body. In general, we call it the Basic Step, and symbolically we call it The Way.

As a fundamental part of this system of movement, this form is related to what you may have learned as a student of Seamm-Jasani. Its applications and objectives will vary now, as seen from the more forceful and solid perspective of Boabom.

First, let us analyze it step by step:

(A) Begin in Osseous Field, your feet together.
(B) Now move to Normal Position, Hands at Your Waist. Bend both your knees, the right more than the left, lifting your right heel while keeping the ball of the foot on the floor. Keep your back straight, pushing your hips just a bit to the back: you will immediately feel tension in the thighs and gluteus.

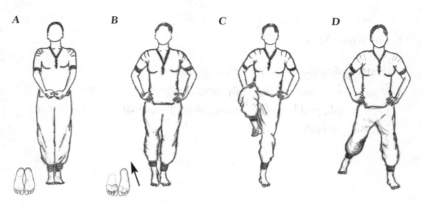

(C) Lift your right foot, with your toes flexed back toward you, inhaling (*nsss . . .*). The sole of your foot should remain aimed at the ground, which is different from the Arched Step, in which the foot is angled to the side.

(D) Exhale (*haaa . . .*) as you bring your foot back down, grazing the floor as it moves back and to the right, following a quarter-circle, as indicated in the drawing.

(E) Finally, you have reached a wide, open position, the right foot back and to the side, just as the drawing shows. Both feet rest parallel to each other, your torso and hips straight, and your weight cen-

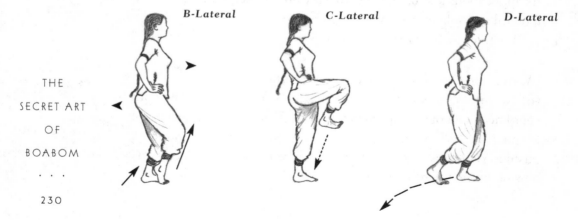

B-Lateral   C-Lateral   D-Lateral

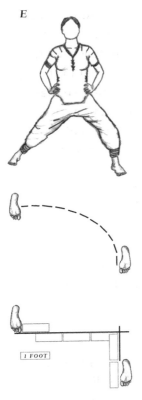

E

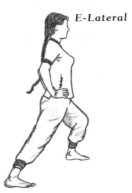

E-Lateral

tered. The distance between the feet should be this: one foot-length back, and three and a half wide (remember that this is measured in the length of your own feet, for we all have different bodies). This gives a solid, general measure that should demand a bit from you; you will immediately feel some tension on the bent leg as well as in the other one, which must be held completely straight, as in the drawing.

(F) To return, keep your hands at your waist and inhale (*nsss . . .*), bend your left leg slightly as you return your right leg to where it began, following the same path but in reverse (D->C->B->A), again tracing a quarter circle. When your right foot has come to the front, pull it up to the height of your knee. Exhale (*haaa . . .*) as you lower your right foot: now both feet are together and you are back where you began, in Osseous Field.

Now practice this same step again, but on the left side. For this, use the exact same movement as developed in letters A through F but in reverse.

This form of step can be seen from many different perspectives. Superficially, someone who knows a bit of fencing can see its essential steps; however, in what we call The Way, you are applying a totally different meaning.

I FOOT

First, the weight of the body should not be moved forward but instead must remain centered, as shown in drawing E: the foot in the back remains hidden and protected, parallel to the front foot, which produces the maximum stretching of the calf muscles, and in this way the lower extremities are prepared for movements that are developed in more advanced stages. The front knee is bent, protecting the left, and casting its protective shadow over the instep. This position is wide, giving you a stronger and more solid base. Farther along in this book you will see that this will allow you to make zigzag movements, which are essential in our Art. When used as a defense projection, this movement can serve (with either a bent or a straight leg) as a terrible lever against the legs of an imaginary opponent. On the other hand, as a step of defense, it does not seek direct and obtuse confrontation, instead searching to flow and elude, teaching to wait and neutralize the possible opponent, instead of confronting with brute force as would two goats or two passionate mentalities (to not say it in another way).

As you practice this step, you can center your imagination in the base of your feet and at the same time on the earth beneath us, to feel the solidity that this position gives us. Imagine yourself an enormous tree with immense, thick roots: nothing can move you from this place! Put your imagination to work!

Remember that it is preferable to practice this Art barefoot. Ideally you can have direct contact with the ground or grass. In this way you can make use of and feed from the magnetic force of the great blue planet . . . believe it or not!

> **Symbolic Name:** The Way
>
> **Initial Position:** Osseous Field
>
> **Breathing:** Inhale (*nsss . . .*) as you raise your foot; exhale (*haaa . . .*) as you bring your foot back and complete the position.
>
> **Duration:** 6 times per side
>
> **Defense Application or Basic Objectives:** Basic step, defense of the anterior leg, form of projection with the posterior leg

16. The Applied Way: Basic Applied Step

After you have come to a basic mastery of the previous step on both sides, you can begin working with this application, as a preparation for the different techniques that are to come.

(A) Begin in Osseous Field, then bring your hands to your waist, lifting your right foot as you inhale (*nsss . . .*): this is the same as the beginning of The Way.

(B) Just as in the previous movement, bring your raised foot back along a quarter circle, exhaling at the same time (*haaa . . .*). Keep your hands at your waist during the entire movement in order to center yourself in this step, which you are trying to learn and cultivate.

A

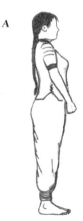 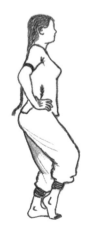

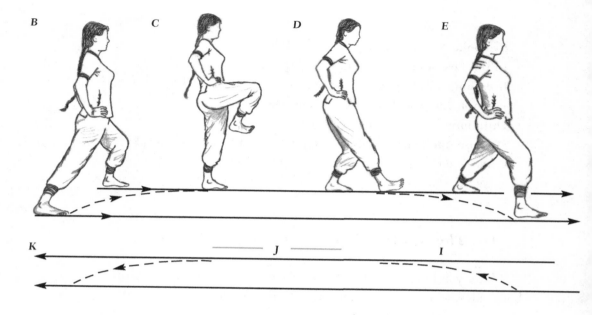

(C) Now inhale (*nsss* . . .), bringing the right foot forward in that same quarter circle, until your foot is at the height of your other knee, in the earlier position.

(D) Immediately continue with the step, but this time moving your foot to the front as you exhale (*haaa* . . .), trying to follow another quarter circle. The path of your foot's descent should be concave, as a bird landing silently on the water.

(E) When you have completed this movement, you have arrived in the same position (The Way) but now with the right foot in front, having traced another full quarter circle.

(F) After two seconds of rest, continue advancing, this time with the left foot coming from behind to be in front. For this, inhale (*nsss* . . .) again, and advance in an arc as before, until your left foot is raised and in front of your right knee.

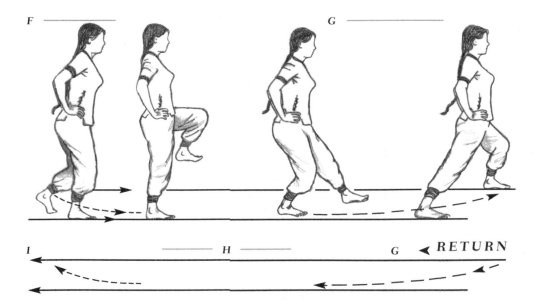

F ——————   G ——————

I ——————— H ———— G ◄ **RETURN**

(G) Exhale (*haaa . . .*) as your foot descends to the front, finishing now in the same position, now with the left forward.

(H) Now we will come back; for this, you must begin by bending your back (right) knee slightly, then immediately bring your left foot back along the first quarter circle. If you look at the drawing, you will see that you must drag your foot along the floor for most of the movement, raising it only at the end while you inhale (*nsss . . .*) and bring it in front of the knee.

(I) Lower your foot now to the back as you exhale (*haaa . . .*), forming the second quarter circle.

(J) Go back one more time, following the same mechanics as before: return with the right leg, bringing it back and inhaling (*nsss . . .*).

(K) Finally, lower your foot to the back as you exhale (*haaa . . .*), and you have returned to the beginning.

BOABOM—THE
TECHNIQUE OF
THE OSSEOUS
ART

. . .

235

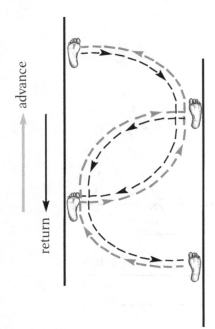

Now you can repeat this entire sequence five times as a way of practicing it, both advancing and coming back. When you have returned to the beginning for the final time, bring your feet together, the right coming to the left, and finish in Osseous Field, just as you began.

This movement should be done solidly and rhythmically once it has been mastered, with a certain speed yet without losing its elegance. As I have mentioned, those who have studied Seamm-Jasani (which works with gentle movements) will have base enough to execute the movements from Boabom with technical precision, yet now with speed, energy, and strength.

This basic step is applied in a zigzag, as you can see in the drawings and especially the patterns of the feet; it might seem like the movement of a snake—evasive, fast, and stealthy.

This exercise, applied as two steps advancing and two returning, is a simple yet efficient practice; besides, you can do it without difficulty in a relatively small space. This two step form is the most fundamental application, for you can also enlarge it to three or four steps, going back in the same number to return to where you began.

Study this movement with attention and care, primarily the first few times you practice it: watch your feet, legs, and trunk, making sure they are in the correct position. This technical precision is very important so that the energy can flow in its proper way and so that you can feel confidence and stability in the application both of this movement and of those to come. Do not worry about reaching a target in front of you or trying to overstretch your body; just look for technical perfection.

Remember to focus your mind on the energy from the feet and legs that travels up through you. Imagine and feel them as solid but flexible branches that, step by step, yield as they simultaneously grasp the ground. Now these branches move the tree, and your body is the firm trunk in this special, living, moving tree.

Symbolic Name: The Applied Way
Initial Position: Osseous Field
Breathing: Inhale (*nsss* . . .) as you raise your foot; exhale (*haaa* . . .) as you bring your foot down, whether forward or back.
Duration: 5 sequences back and forth
Defense Application or Basic Objectives: Practice of the basic step, as well as a zigzag defense

---

Common Mistakes

In both The Way and The Applied Way, a common mistake is an imbalanced trunk, whether to the front, trying to gain distance, or to the back.

Another common error is to open the back foot, which generally happens because keeping the feet parallel requires a lot of work from the calf muscles. Try to correct the feet, keeping them aligned (like the tires of a car!).

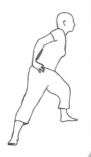

17. The Way and the Force of the Spiral: Basic Step and Individual Projection

By the time you have reached this movement, you should have acquired a certain skill with the previous movements; thus, we will begin developing each basic step in combination with The Applied Way (technique number 16), creating different coordinations.

This will be the first basic union between steps and hand techniques. It is executed in the following way:

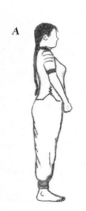

(A) Osseous Field

(B) Immediately move to Normal Position, Hands at Your Waist.

(C) Lift your right foot as you inhale (*nsss . . .*), and bring it to the back as you exhale (*haaa . . .*), just as in The Way (number 15). Now bring your hands into The Fist That Is Born, but this time on the other side, with your left hand in a fist and your right hand open, in front of your sternum.

(D) Project your left fist as you inhale (*nsss . . .*) as in The Force of the Spiral (technique number 6).

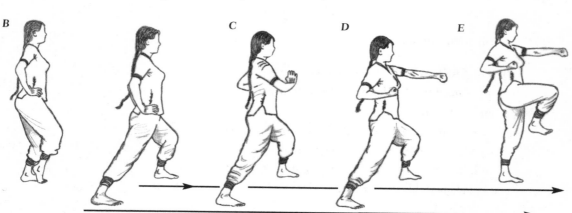

(E) Advancing with your right foot, trace a semicircle as you did in The Applied Way, while keeping your hand in the exact same position (do not move it!). You should exhale through this entire step, from takeoff to landing.

(F) Finish exhaling as your right foot comes to rest in front; you will notice that in this coordination the exhalation is enlarged, adapted to the entire step. The step must be quick and the breathing sharp, although without losing the technique. Remember that you must keep your arm in the same position.

(G) Once you are in the new position, project your right fist to the front, inhaling (*nsss . . .*) and generating as much power as possible. The movement must be precise, with its force centered in the arm. Do not move your shoulders or curve your back. It does not matter if the movement seems short: the objective is not distance but technique, control over your body, and control over yourself! Focus your mind on that; the power and speed will be born naturally.

(H) Continue advancing but now with the left foot moving forward.

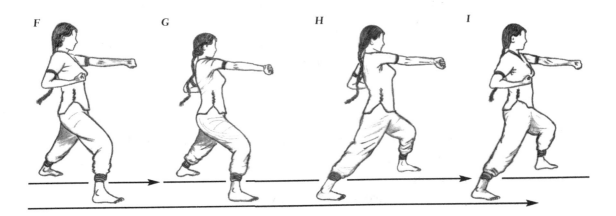

F   G   H   I

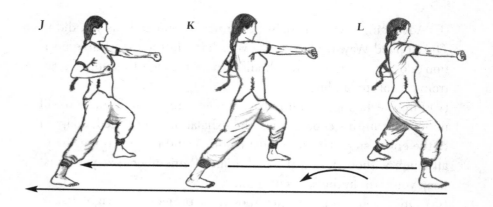

Exhale completely (*haaa* . . .), keeping the right arm rigid through the entire movement.

(I) When you are still, rest for two seconds, then project the left fist in The Force of the Spiral, with certainty, as you inhale (*nsss!*).

Now you can begin the process of returning, following the same mechanism.

(J) The left foot ascends and descends to the back as you exhale (*haaa* . . .).

(K) As soon as you reach this position, project the right arm as you inhale (*nsss!*).

(L) Go back a second time, following the same movement, but now with the right foot going back as you exhale (*haaa* . . .); the arm remains still.

Now you are back where you began.

You can repeat this whole cycle three more times, beginning again with the projection of the right arm (D). You do not need to return to The Fist That Is Born.

Once you have finished all of your repetitions, bring your hands

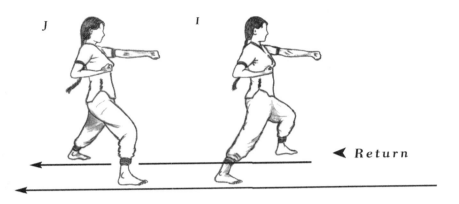

J   I

◄ Return

to your waist and bringing your right foot forward, place it next to the left, finishing in Osseous Field.

This is a basic form of coordination, but it must be executed properly: the development of all the subsequent coordinations will depend on how you practice and come to understand this movement. Besides, it will shape your discipline and concentration, your capacity to focus on the technique itself, and your capacity to individualize the energy developed from the legs and trunk to the arms.

In the subsequent movements, you will continue with this same kind of work but using different hand techniques. If you are careful, you will see that in all the coordinations of this kind, the steps and projections are isolated; they work in this way in order to precisely develop the technique, without hurrying from one piece to the next.

NOTE: When you have had spent a good amount of time with this movement, you should be able to dispose of the step by step form in which we have organized this technique. Thus each step can be executed simultaneously with the projection of the arms, which should finish its motion at the same time as the foot comes to rest.

When executing this united technique, the inhalation and exhalation should work in conjunction with the movement; thus you would inhale as you began your advance (D, E), and exhale as your foot descends, at the same time projecting your arm (F, G). This doubles the power: the step together with the arm in its spiral, or whichever projection corresponds.

For now, continue with the basic application (step by step) as it has been described, and leave the more complex applications for later work.

Common Mistakes

In this drawing you can see clearly how the body has moved forward, following the impulse of the arm. This mistake is common not only in this exercise but also in the following ones, which combine steps and projections.

Another technical mistake is not twisting the fist as corresponds with the movement: the twisting causes a tension in the arm, shoulder, and trunk that increases with the step, but it is important to persevere through this challenge in order to master the technique, rather than falling into the mistake shown in the drawing.

Also, bending the rear leg will remove stability and solidity from the step.

> **Symbolic Name:** The Way and the Force of the Spiral
>
> **Initial Position:** Osseous Field and The Way
>
> **Breathing:** Inhale (*nsss . . .*) when projecting the hand; exhale (*haaa . . .*) with the step.
>
> **Duration:** 3 times forward and back
>
> **Defense Application or Basic Objectives:** Basic middle projection in conjunction with the step (to the stomach or sternum). The use of multiple forces in motion: the base of the position and the energy of the step; the solidity of the trunk; the power of the arm in its projection, its spiral shape, its final twist (applied with the Twin Mountains), the force generated by the opposite arm, with its elbow pulled back.

18. The Way and the Force of the Double Spiral: Basic Step and Double Projection

Now we will use the same process, only this time applied to the double spiral movement. This is usually a strong and continuous application. Use the same pattern as in the previous movement (17). Begin in Osseous Field with The Way with The Solid Fist (A). Project the Force of the Double Spiral (B) while inhaling; then, as you advance, exhale and contract your arms so that when you reach the final position they have returned to The Solid Fist. Project again while inhaling, then advance for the second time. Apply the same pattern when going back.

When you have finished moving, you will be back where you began.

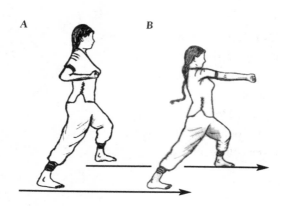

A   B

To practice the movement, repeat the entire sequence three times.

Once you have returned to starting position, bring your feet together and finish in Osseous Field.

Symbolic Name: The Way and the Force of the Double Spiral
Initial Position: Osseous Field and The Way
Breathing: Inhale (*nsss*) when projecting the fists; exhale (*haaa*) with the step.
Duration: 3 times through the complete sequence
Defense Application or Basic Objectives: Double midlevel projection in union with the steps; technical defense against larger opponents

19. The Way and the Essential Low Block: Basic Step and Low Block

We will now develop a similar coordination, this time using the Essential Low Block. We will use the same movement and breathing as in movement 17, only this time applied to the Essential Low Block.

A–B   C 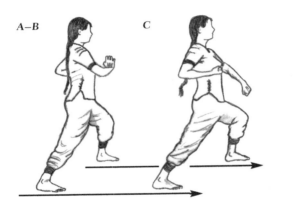   C-Frontal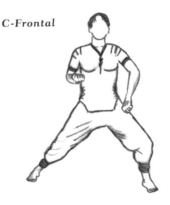

Symbolic Name: The Way and the Essential Low Block

Initial Position: Osseous Field and The Way

Breathing: Inhale (*nsss . . .*) when projecting the hand; exhale (*haaa . . .*) with the step.

Duration: 3 times forward and back

Defense Application or Basic Objectives: Defense of the low zone, mainly the thigh, or use of the movement as a projection to the opponent's low zone in conjunction with the step

BOABOM—THE
TECHNIQUE OF
THE OSSEOUS
ART

. . .

245

20. The Way and the Bond of Rectitude: Basic Step and Crossed High Block

This time we apply the idea from movement 18, both for the two steps forward and for the steps back; only now we will use The Bond of Rectitude.

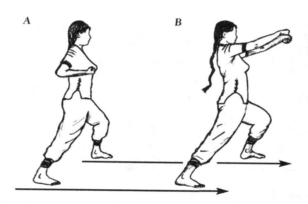

Symbolic Name: The Way and the Bond of Rectitude

Initial Position: Osseous Field and The Way

Breathing: Inhale (*nsss . . .*) when projecting the hands; exhale (*haaa . . .*) with the step.

Duration: 3 times forward and back

Defense Application or Basic Objectives: High projection (generally to the face) or high blocking (against descending strikes) in conjunction with the steps, in order to achieve the maximum power when advancing and efficiency when returning

21. The Way and the Open Spiral: Basic Step and Individual Circular Projection of the Palm

Apply the same technique as in movement 17, this time using The Force of the Spiral.

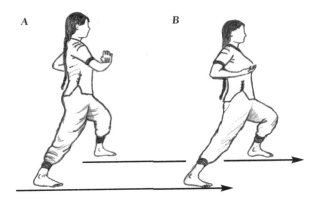

Symbolic Name: The Way and the Open Spiral

Initial Position: Osseous Field and The Way

Breathing: Inhale (*nsss . . .*) when projecting the hand; exhale (*haaa . . .*) with the step.

Duration: 3 times back and forth

Defense Application or Basic Objectives: Midlevel open projection (to the sternum or stomach), which moves a maximum of energy when combined with the step

BOABOM—THE
TECHNIQUE OF
THE OSSEOUS
ART

. . .

247

22. The Way and the Open Double Spiral: Basic Step and Double Circular Projection of the Palm

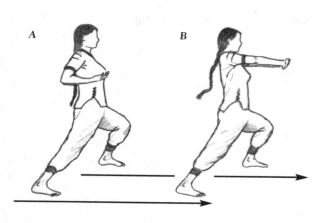

In this movement we will apply the same coordinative and respiratory work from movement 18, now using The Force of the Double Spiral.

> **Symbolic Name:** The Way and the Open Double Spiral
> **Initial Position:** Osseous Field and The Way
> **Breathing:** Inhale (*nsss . . .*) when projecting the hands; exhale (*haaa . . .*) with the step.
> **Duration:** 3 times forward and back
> **Defense Application or Basic Objectives:** Open double midlevel projection with step; with this combination, you create an unstoppable form of projection, providing a great energy and power over short distances.

Stage IV. Initial Foot Techniques

23. The Whip Foot—Middle

We will continue the learning process by focusing on various movements of foot projections: you will see the simplest and most basic forms, for we are continuing to follow the idea of this book, which is introducing the beginning student to Boabom in a practical way, covering the most essential techniques in as detailed a way as possible. Remember that a good foundation makes a good building; if you understand well what has been developed in this book, then your future learning, whether through another book on this Art or directly through one of our schools, will be much easier for you, and you will be able to advance quickly, having had a strong technical foundation.

Many people believe that they can learn everything from a book. I do not wish to disappoint them, but that belief is very far from reality: it would be like pretending to be a doctor after having read one book on biology. More realistically, we can try to make this book a good introduction to our Art, and with a bit of practice in the first movements, you can prepare to learn the great Art that you can know . . . if you really want to . . . if you are prepared to look for it.

We will now move into the basic techniques of foot projection, which we will symbolically call The Whip Foot. Pay careful attention to the details, for this movement has many of them, despite its apparently simple appearance.

Follow the instructions step-by-step at first, then apply them in a more fluid, spontaneous way.

BOABOM—THE
TECHNIQUE OF
THE OSSEOUS
ART

. . .

249

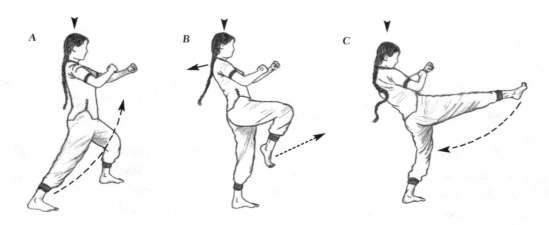

Begin, as in every technique, in Osseous Field.

Bring your hands to your waist, inhale (*nsss* . . .), and exhale (*haaa* . . .), bringing your right foot back as you execute The Way, which will be the first technical foundation of this movement.

(A) Immediately form the Medium Block (technique number 14) with your hands, inhaling (*nsss!*) and exhaling (*haaa!*). The left hand is first crossed behind the vertically held right hand and then moves to the front, where it remains, in front of the right. Now we have the complete base and initial position for our foot movement: feet in The Way and hands in Medium Block, the left slightly in front of the right. We will always begin from and return to this position in this technique and the two that follow: it will be our support.

Stage of Projection:
(B) You will now project with your right foot, which begins in the back. The hands will remain where they are, serving as a basic defense and support for the execution of the movement. First, raise your right foot to the center (in the same quarter circle that I have

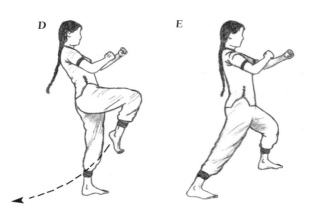

D   E

mentioned before), keeping your back straight. The ascent of the foot imitates the stepping movements, but with the difference that the raised foot points downward and the toes are flexed back toward you, up and away from the floor; see the drawing for details. In conjunction with this, begin by inhaling (*nsss . . .*).

(C) With the foot already risen, project it forward, sinking it into the midzone. The foot should be pointed forward (in plantar flexion), but with the toes pointed back toward you. The contact of the strike should be made only with the ball of the foot, *not* with the toes or instep. At the same time as you project your foot, you should lean back slightly, using the hips as your axis, to give more strength and penetration to the movement. Try to imitate the posture shown in the drawing.

NOTE: Obviously, owing to the nature of this movement, I am detailing the process step-by-step, but in practice the idea is that this movement is fluid and moves quickly back and forth.

(D) Immediately, like a whip, contract your leg, bringing your foot back, next to the opposite knee. It is here that you finish inhaling.

There should be almost no delay between the projection and retraction described in C and D above: it should be like a spark, a quick movement, precise and with great energy. Remember that the force and power of Boabom lies in its speed, not in its weight or strength.

(E) Now bring the foot back, exhaling (*haaa . . .*) as we return to The Way. Repeat this whole process so that the whole motion of raising the foot, projecting it, and bringing it back is as fast as possible while you still care for the technique, never losing its precision. Resting a moment between projections, repeat this process ten more times.

When you have finished this, to rest, bring your hands to your waist and gather your feet (right to left) into Osseous Field. From this position, return to the beginning of this movement and execute it again, but this time on the left side, with the left leg.

This movement, when well done, is incredibly effective in its speed, reach, and power. It produces a triple effect: the force of the projection itself, the strike with the ball of the foot (which is naturally a very hard region), and finally, the body as a kind of scale or balance, which delivers more power to the hips. The union of this movement has a great energy, and thus the objective is for you to first learn the process well, and later to do it with speed, like a spark. Only in this way will you understand the movement.

Be patient and you will feel why we have called it, symbolically, The Whip Foot. If you experience some difficulty trying to flex your toes back at the same time as you are projecting your foot forward, do not worry, for it is a bit complex at first, though with time you will be able to do it.

This kind of movement is very efficient as a form of defense, because it unites speed and force in a relatively simple application. As for the psychical or meditative development, you must imagine that the latent energy is centered in the ball of the foot, but that this descends from the trunk, hip, and gluteus: these are like the opposite pole, which, when connected with the foot through this movement, cause a strong current to arc through the leg.

Common Mistakes

The first common mistake is in swinging the leg straight to the
front without first bending it. This reduces the effectiveness of the
movement.

Bending the back forward shortens the posterior muscles of the
thigh, which makes the projection of the leg to the front impossible, or at least very clumsy.

Bending the toes down, and thus causing them to be the principal
point of impact, is also a serious mistake. If this was done in real application, it would
surely cause self-injury.

NOTE: These same mistakes should be considered for the two subsequent techniques,
numbers 24 and 25.

Symbolic Name: The Whip Foot—Middle
Initial Position: Osseous Field and The Way
Breathing: Inhale through the projection and retraction of the
leg (*nsss!*); exhale (*haaa . . .*) when returning to the initial
position.
Duration: 10 times on each side
Defense Application or Basic Objectives: Middle projection of
the foot to the thorax or genital area

BOABOM—THE

TECHNIQUE OF

THE OSSEOUS

ART

. . .

253

24. The Whip Foot—Low:
Foot Projection—Low

We will now form the same projection of the foot but to the low zone. Follow these movements step by step:

Begin in Osseous Field.

Bring your hands to your waist, inhale (*nsss . . .*) and exhale (*haaa . . .*), moving your right foot back into the Basic Step.

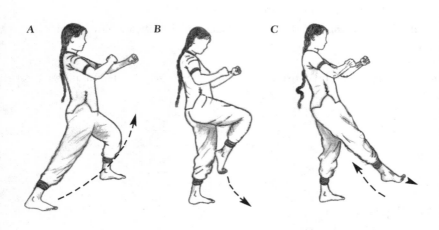

(A) Bring the hands to the Medium Block, inhaling and exhaling as you would normally with this movement. End with the left hand in front.

(B) To project the right foot, first lift it to the center as you begin inhaling (*nsss . . .*), keeping your arms still.

(C) Project your right foot to the front as in the previous movement, but this time aiming low, coming close to but not touching the floor. Remember to keep your toes bent back, as the contact of this strike must be produced with the ball of the foot.

Like a whip, retract your foot quickly, bringing it back, bent now, to its high point, the foot at knee level. Your inhalation should end here.

Bring this foot back into The Way, exhaling (*haaa . . .*).

You have now returned to the Basic Step, the hands never having moved from their basic guard.

Repeat this complete process ten more times.

When you are done with this, bring your hands to your waist and close to Osseous Field. Now you can work with the left side.

This movement may seem strange in the way that the foot is directed low. In its defensive form, Boabom has as its objectives very precise weak points, so it extends no defense in an unnecessary direction; thus, in this movement, the objective can be the instep (quite a delicate zone) of an imaginary opponent. But I wish to remind you, again, that all of this is I-M-A-G-I-N-A-R-Y and not about walking around and practicing on the first person you see. If you do, you will prove that you have not understood this book at all, and that it would have been much better for you to have purchased some kind of commando manual, which I imagine must be quite common and very, very cheap.

Simply dedicate yourself to use this Art as a way to focus your mind, giving it discipline as you awaken your energy in a positive way and for a positive reason—for looking within!

Symbolic Name: The Whip Foot—Low

Initial Position: Osseous Field and The Way

Breathing: Inhale through the projection and retraction of the leg (*nsss!*); exhale (*haaa . . .*) when returning to the initial position.

Duration: 10 times on each side

Defense Application or Basic Objectives: Low projection of the foot, generally to the instep or patella

25. The Whip Foot—High:
Foot Projection—High

The next movement comes from the others, but this has a high projection, which is a bit more complex.

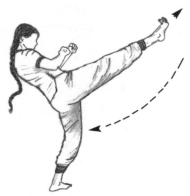

Begin in Osseous Field, and continue with the normal process: hands to waist, inhale (*nsss!*) and exhale (*haaa . . .*) as you move your right foot back into The Way.

Bring your hands to the Medium Block, inhaling and exhaling. The left hand prevails in front.

As usual, to project the right foot, lift it to the center as you begin the work of inhalation (*nsss . . .*).

Project your right foot up high now, toward the neck or head of an imaginary opponent. Your foot should be aimed diagonally upward as your trunk leans slightly back, helping you to balance. As in the other movements, the contact of the strike is with the ball of the foot, so pay attention to the drawing and the direction of your toes.

Retract your foot, again quickly, like a whip, bringing it back to the level of the other knee. Here ends the inhalation.

Return with this same foot to The Way as you exhale (*haaa . . .*). Through the whole movement, the hands have not moved.

Repeat this process ten times.

At the end, to rest, bring your hands to your waist, gather the right foot to the left as you would when closing The Way, and return to Osseous Field. As in the other techniques, you can now work with the left side.

This foot movement is a bit more complex, as it requires more flexibility in the leg to reach the desired height; if you have done a good preparatory Jass-U, however, you should not have any problems. But please do not be confused: when I say "high," I do not mean that you must have a fantastic elasticity like the main characters in many movies, who seem to be made out of rubber. These kinds of gymnastic stretches are completely unnecessary, both from the perspective of an effective defense and from the positive energy we might achieve. If security and psychical force were in proportion to our stretching, then it would be a simple matter to solve . . . but to the disappointment of many, it just is not so. Therefore, work patiently, and at your own measure. The main idea is that this movement has its whiplike effect, that is, going back and forth quickly with the foot: with time you will increase its height.

Symbolic Name: The Whip Foot—High

Initial Position: Osseous Field and The Way

Breathing: Inhale through the projection and retraction of the leg (*nsss!*); exhale (*haaa . . .*) when returning to the initial position.

Duration: 10 times on each side

Defense Application or Basic Objectives: High projection of the foot; its objectives will be the neck and head.

Stage V. Study of the Forms of Reaction

The complete development of this stage is treated separately in chapter 4, since it requires both special attention and a certain maturity within these movements before it can be well understood and properly executed. In order to know when to begin learning each of the Forms of Reaction, study the Pedagogical Chart on page 133.

In order to avoid confusion in the sequence of the final class, the movements in chapter 4 are numbered 26 to 31.

Stage VI. Meditation and Closing the Class

Breathing Technique of The Inner Power

Always, when closing the class, we will apply the Breathing Technique of The Inner Power twice (see chapter 2, exercise 5, for details).

After this you can sit down and relax for a few moments.

With this you have completed this cycle of our teaching. Try to be precise and careful in your study, and review each section whenever you have any doubt as to the details of the movements developed within them. It may be that, on first reading, they seem simple, but in practice each and every one of these techniques has many elements to which you must pay attention.

In the next chapter we will also see a stage of closing meditation, which will seal the teaching developed in this book.

Chapter 4

BOABOM—THE FORMS OF REACTION

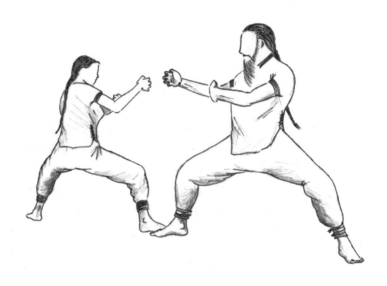

*The force of the lever, the inevitable inertia, the confusion of the spiral,
the power of rectitude, and the surprise of velocity
are the threads of the Art in practice . . .*

*—Grupta, The Constructor,
from* The Legend of the Mmulmmat

COMPLEMENTARY STAGES
OF THE CLASS

Stage V. Study of the Forms of Reaction

In this stage you will develop what, in Boabom, we call reactions or reflexes: all of this cycle forms a more complex complement within the general development of a class. You will also notice that we have continued with the same numbering as in the previous chapter, for these and those together belong to one whole unified system.

In this stage you will see that we will form short coordinations that will unite breathing, steps, blocks, and projections of the hands and feet. The main objective of these exercises is to simulate, or imagine, ourselves before an imaginary opponent (remember: imaginary!), which will help us to measure and develop our capacity for reflection, decision, confidence, speed-coordination, and, in summary, internal-external energy.

These forms are divided into two parts:

1. Reactions to Projections (or strikes)
2. Reactions to Being Taken or Grabbed

Both forms of reaction seem to be simple and basic systems, but they require study and understanding beyond their apparent simplicity. Remember that these coordinations will form an applied continuation of the techniques you have already learned and that if you have practiced those carefully, these will be much easier to understand.

Every person has a natural and normal fear of being violently grabbed or taken; even more, there are cases in which this natural fear has been increased by traumatic experiences those people have lived. One of the objectives of this stage is as a practical way to improve upon those weaknesses and to see life from a more positive perspective (which is always useful to all of us). From this perspective we can see that this practice has multiple purposes: we can use it externally, as a form of defense (which is the external, or superficial, part), but we can also use it to improve our own self-control, to go beyond our fears to where we can finally cultivate security and spontaneity in our thoughts. All of these physical elements knit and strengthen the weave of our defense and magnetic field.

Each Form of Reaction will have a beginning, an action, and a development or reaction, which is the technique itself. You will always begin in the Osseous Field position (chapter 3, technique 1), which will then change into an initial position, depending on the coordination itself. In the three forms of Reaction to Projections, the imaginary opponent will project a basic movement of the fist, which can be used as a reference. In the three forms of Reactions to Being Taken, we will show where and how the imaginary opponent would grab you.

In this stage Boabom comes to life as an Art of Defense; however, and I cannot insist on this enough times, its real goal goes far beyond simple defense. The idea is to delve deep into the mechanism of the mind, its coordinative capacity, and its ability to react before different stimuli, thus turning all its potential into fluent technique and effective reaction. To us, it is a form of meditation, of channeling the physical-psychical energies; if the mind and body are not capable of acting together, their reactions, both physical and psychological, tend to be clumsy, and even more so in situations of pressure, whether external or of panic. But do not worry, for everything can be developed.

When you study these reactions, try to isolate yourself as best you can from the world that surrounds you; focus and you will see that you will simultaneously rest from your daily problems and feel renewed, that you have unloaded your negative thoughts and will be better able to continue your work and life with a better disposition.

Finally, and though it may sound strange or contradictory, these simple coordinations will help you to think spontaneously, beyond reason, and to discover your instinct. But be careful! I mean the real instinct, the one that is noble, kind, confident in its actions, and without external ambition. I am explaining this because more than one person could use these words as a justification of even more stupidities than they already may have committed in their lives. It is easy to confuse Art of Defense with Martial Method, or acting with a pure mind with acting by camouflaged interests, or even seeking instinct with finding justifications for our frustrated desires. Thus take this stage in its proper meaning: as an exercise beyond any apparent defense it might produce. See it as a meditation, to focus your mind, and with that to search for awakening the nobility and the true I: quiet and with all of its power liberated.

26. Form of Reaction to Projection— Number 1: The Efficiency of Simplicity

All of these forms of reaction to strikes must begin with a meditative-imaginary task: you must form your opponent in front of you, and upon this opponent you will apply the technique without causing anyone any harm. In general, your imaginary partner will have the task of projecting a technique toward a specific point of your body, and this is the point you will have to defend: your opponent's projection will always be the Basic Step with the Force of the Spiral (technique number 17), which we assume our opponent will be doing with speed and energy (taking the step and projecting at the same time). Try to see this opponent not as an enemy but as a virtual assistant who is advising you in your physical-psychical exertions, through which you are giving life (and a spark!) to Boabom.

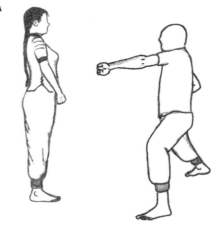

A

In the drawing, you can see the student facing the imaginary opponent, waiting, ready to step forward and begin the action-reaction that forms this coordination.

The first form of reaction will be simple, strong, and direct. Your imaginary opponent will use a hand projection directed toward your lower zone, and you must react with precision and technique. With time you will discover the spontaneous velocity that is a fundamental element in our Art.

For this, the first form of reaction, follow this order of movements:

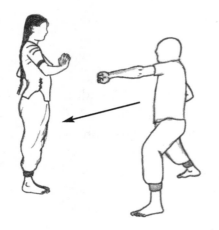

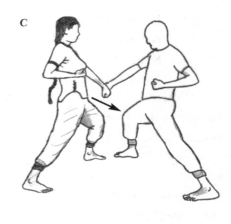

(A) Begin in Osseous Field.

(B) In this same position, with the feet remaining together, form The Fist That Is Born. It will serve us as a beginning.

(C) *Action:* Your imaginary opponent, who is in front of you, will step forward and project his hand toward your low zone, moving with decision and speed.

Reaction: Immediately step back with your right foot, The Way. Move your hands in the same time in the Basic Low Block, protecting the threatened area (for details, see technique number 19). Inhale as you lift your leg (*nsss . . .*) and exhale as you step back simultaneously with your Low Block (*haaa!*). As you can see, you have combined the step, the hand technique, and the breathing all in an instant. The strike has been annuled.

(D) Immediately after blocking, pull your left fist back as you advance with your right leg in The Applied Way, inhaling (*nsss . . .*). At the same time as your foot reaches its goal, project your right fist down (The Force of the Spiral, Low), directed below your opponent's belly button, though not too low. Exhale in unison with this

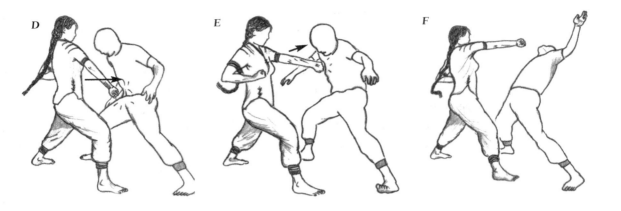

D   E   F

projection (*haaa!*). This will cause your opponent to bend forward, surprised.

(E) Immediately project The Force of the Spiral with your left hand to the middle zone, just below the sternum, inhaling (*nsss!*), causing our virtual assistant to bend farther to the front.

(F) Now project The Force of the Spiral high, using your right hand. Exhale (*haaa!*) as the impact is entirely in your opponent's face.

The objective is for this sequence of projections (low, middle, high) to be quick and continuous, one after the other without stopping. When well executed, this sequence will seem to occur without hesitation, and when it has been perfected, it will look as if you have projected three arms at once! The discharge of energy will be unstoppable.

Return now to your back leg (right joining left), bringing your feet together. Go now to Osseous Field as a technical way of ending this coordination and to prove that your efforts are disciplined and complete.

As you can see, this form unites the breathing technique in a particular way, accompanying the movement in order to give it the maximum speed and precision. At the same time, the step acts as a low defense, and united with the block of the hand, it is unbreakable. Finally, the immediate projection to the front combined with the step reverses the action with a series of projections that must be quick to be effective: low, medium, and finally high, which has a great effect, for, as can be appreciated, the opponent tends to bend as a consequence of the previous movements. We have executed a forceful reaction that can easily disarm our imaginary opponent, whatever his or her size.

Use your imagination, live the action, and feel the energy that unites the body-mind.

Symbolic Name: The Efficiency of Simplicity
Initial Position: Osseous Field
Steps Within the Movement: 4 (4 seconds each)
Zone Defended: Low zone: genital area or thigh
Technical and Respiratory Development (S=Step):
Osseous Field into The Fist That Is Born
  S1. Right Basic Step with Low Blocking. Inhale and exhale (*nsss . . . haaa . . .*).
  S2. Advance the right foot with the Low Force of the Spiral, right hand. Inhale (*nsss . . .*) and exhale (*haaa!*).
  S3. Middle Force of the Spiral, left hand. Inhale (*nsss!*).
  S4. High Force of the Spiral, right hand. Exhale (*haaa!*).

27. Form of Reaction to Projection— Number 2: The Spark of Opposing Forces

You will now learn the second reaction: do not try to execute it if you have not understood the previous one. Take some time to digest the idea, which can actually take many sessions of review. Remember that the best way is to follow the Pedagogical Chart on page 133.

The sequence is as follows:

(A) Begin in Osseous Field (see movement 26).
(B) *Action:* The imaginary opponent is in front of you and begins the action by stepping forward and projecting the hand to your middle zone.
Reaction: The response begins: open the left foot to the side in the Universal Position, Arched Step, but when lifting your foot, bring your hands directly from Osseous Field upward, crossing them in the first part of the Middle Block, protecting your right lateral zone. Inhale with this (*nsss!*).

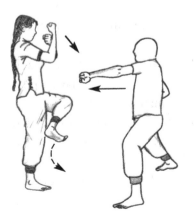
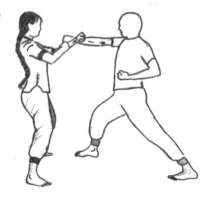

(C) At the exact same time as your left foot lands to form Universal Position, bring your hands in front of you in the Middle Block, with your left hand in front, directly blocking the arm of our imaginary opponent out and away. All this is executed in one movement, tied to one exhalation (*haaa!*).

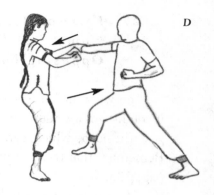

D

(D) Grab, with your left hand, the arm you have just blocked.

(E) Pull your opponent strongly toward you at the same time as you begin The Whip Foot by lifting your knee. Inhale (*nsss!*).

(F) Project The Whip Foot to the middle of your opponent's body as you exhale (*haaa!*); the impact produced by the opposing forces of the body pulled forward and the strike of the foot can be of an incredible power.

Return now, your right foot joining your left, and with your feet together, come back to Osseous Field.

In this form of reaction we have new elements that make the coordination more complex. One is uniting the Medium Block and the Arched Step with a complete breathing; the other is blocking and pulling the arm or wrist of the opponent toward us. If well executed, this type of reaction is highly effective.

Live your mind in your entire body, for here you will need each link to act in a coordinated and fluid manner in order to have a positive achievement. Imagine that the opposing force comes straight at you, but as tends to happen in life, you must risk, daring to take all of that energy directly, knowing how to confront it with confidence and thus to solve the problem once and for all.

Remember that the main idea, as in all of Boabom, is never hav-

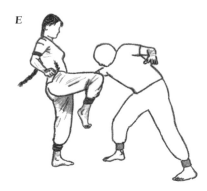 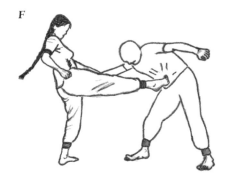

ing to use this kind of technique on another person, keeping it only as a conductor of discipline, concentration, meditation, and expansion of our energy in a positive way.

Symbolic Name: The Spark of Opposing Forces
Initial Position: Osseous Field
Steps Within the Movement: 3 (4 seconds each)
Zone Defended: Middle-high zone: solar plexus, chest, or chin
Technical and Respiratory Development (S=Step):

Osseous Field

S1. Left Arched Step with Medium Block. Inhale and exhale (*nsss! haaa!*).

S2. Grab with your left hand. Inhale (*nsss . . .*).

S3. Pull opponent toward you, and right Middle Whip Foot. Exhale (*haaa!*).

Osseous Field

28. Form of Reaction to Projection—Number 3: The Force of Two

We will now develop a third reaction, this time protecting the general high zone from a direct projection (as shown in the drawings), a descending strike, or an attack with a stick or similar weapon.

The development is as follows:

(A) Begin in Osseous Field (see Movement 26).
(B) *Action:* Our imaginary opponent is facing us and will be projecting the hand technique toward our high zone (neck or head).
Reaction: The reaction begins by taking the hands into The Solid Fist.
(C) In a quick response, and once your opponent is already upon you, step back in the Basic Step with your right foot, gaining distance. At the same time, project to the front with the Crossed High Block (The Bond of Rectitude), forming a mass of great power that protects the whole head. Inhale through this whole action (*nsss!*).

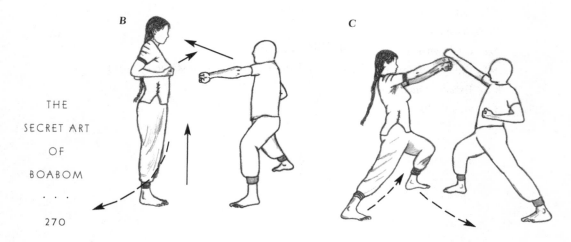

(D) Advance immediately with your right leg, at the same time contracting both arms into the Solid Fist. Here begins the exhalation.

(E) As your right leg reaches the ground, project the Double Force of the Spiral and complete your exhalation (*haaa!*).

Go back now, left foot to right, and return to where you began, finishing in Osseous Field.

You have projected a solid reaction of immense power, since both the left and right have acted together symmetrically, both as a defense and as a projection.

In this movement you can distinguish how inhalation and exhalation leave their normal pattern of application and are joined in a way that produces a quicker and more continuous movement. As for the block, the detailed drawing will give you a clearer idea of the impact that it should produce, not only stopping and deflecting the action but also causing deep pain in the arm of the imaginary opponent.

With this, you have completed the coordinative stage of action and reaction.

D

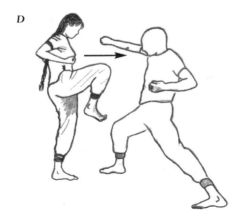

E

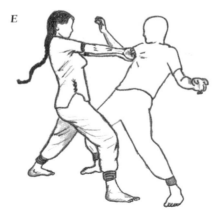

29. Form of Reaction to Being Taken— Number 1: The Ineffable Double Spiral

This is the first of the second kind of reaction, which is in response to being grabbed or taken. Here you will continue your study of basic ways to react, but now our imaginary opponent or virtual assistant has seized some part of our body. In these cases, part of our reaction is the way in which we can release ourselves in a technical, clean, and effective way, at the same time as we reverse the opponent's grip. We measure here our capacity of reaction when we feel the weight of another force upon us, not letting ourselves be intimidated by that weight.

In each of these coordinations we will use a specific technique to show where we are being grabbed, thus creating a discipline to the movement while simulating the opponent's actual grasp. This tech-

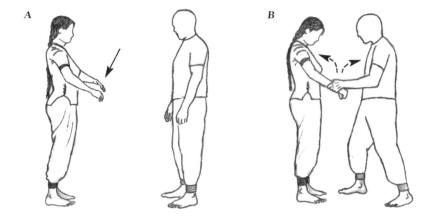

nique will be applied as two gentle taps, with one or both hands, indicating the precise location of contact. This will immediately bring the attention of your mind to the point of immediate interest.

Now we will move to the practice of the first of these three forms of reaction: here we will use the wrists together in reaction.

(A) Begin the coordination by standing in the Base Position (chapter 1, exercise 1), feet separated slightly, hands in front of you, and indicate with two short slaps, one to each hand, that both of your wrists will be seized. Now you are ready for the action.

(B) *Action:* Your imaginary opponent is in front of you, violently taking you by both wrists. Your opponent is big, and he thinks he is even bigger (but do not worry, for he who thinks himself big is only physically big, but not psychically so!).

(C) *Reaction:* In one movement, you will quickly twist both of your forearms and wrists so that your palms finish facing upward, at the same time inhaling (*nsss!*) and bending your knees, lifting the right foot a bit more, as if you were beginning The Way.

C 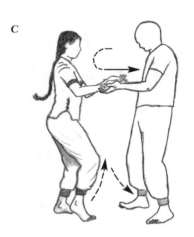 D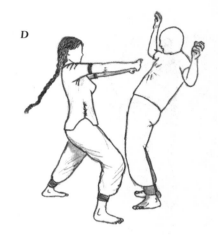

(D) Again, in one impulse, advance in The Applied Way, with the right foot stepping forward. Project at the same time with both hands in the Double Open Spiral, striking your imaginary opponent in the chest. Through this we exhale (*haaa!*), discharging all of our power.

Return now (right joining left) to where you began, with your feet together. Go to Osseous Field as a technical way of ending the action.

As you may have seen, we have used a form of freeing ourselves that is very simple, but highly effective if well executed. This teaches us that mind is far superior to strength (though it is a shame that those with a mind are too often in service to those with strength, but that is another story).

There are three factors, working here in unison, which together produce an effective liberation: the quick twist of the wrists (like an explosion); the inhalation and bending of the knees, which brings tension to the trunk in general; and the immediate advance and projection of the open hands, which completes our total liberation, combined with an effective and firm defense over a short distance. A real opponent would easily be thrown back.

Use your imagination and feel your forearms and hands full of a great energy, moving with both speed and power.

Symbolic Name: The Ineffable Double Spiral

Initial Position: Base Position

Steps Within the Movement: 2 (3 seconds)

Zone Taken: Both hands, taken at the wrists

Technical and Respiratory Development (S=Step): Base Position, with two light slaps on the wrists

    S1. Turn the hands. Inhale (*nsss!*).

    S2. Advance with your right foot in the Basic Step and project the Open Double Spiral. Exhale (*haaa!*).

    Osseous Field

---

30. Form of Reaction to Being Taken—
Number 2: The Fish That Escapes

This, the next form of reaction, is very direct. This time our imaginary opponent is a little more bold and has approached from the back, holding us with both arms, trusting his surprise and strength. Our form for releasing ourselves from this is simple, but it requires attention and decisiveness!

(A) Begin in Base Position, the legs slightly separated. At the same time, indicate with two gentle taps to the sides of your arms where your imaginary opponent's grasp will make contact with your body. You are ready now for the action and reaction.

(B) *Action:* You are taken from behind with a strong hug.

(C) *Reaction:* You must simultaneously bend both knees (the right more so, lifting your heel as in The Way) as you project the Force of the Double Spiral forward. Inhale (*nsss!*).

(D) In this drawing you should notice the projection of both fists in

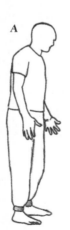
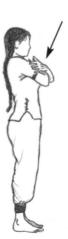
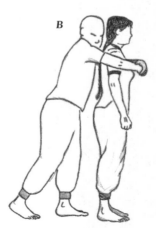

a complete Double Spiral. If you execute this movement well, though it may be simple, you will be immediately released.

(E) Now you must use the force of reaction, which is completed with the retraction of the Double Spiral: your arms rush back to your sides, your hands in fists, and both elbows project directly behind you, a strong element that will easily throw our imaginary opponent back. Exhale through this movement (*haaa!*).

To finish, bring your feet back together and move into Osseous Field.

This is an effective reaction, which can be applied if ever it is needed. Another good thing about Boabom is that while it helps us to know ourselves and gives us vitality, at the same time it can be used to defend us if we ever need it (though the goal may be different). Freeing yourself from the hug is produced by a triple effort that must be united into one simultaneous movement in order to be totally effective: lowering the body, combined with the force of the rising arms as they turn and project forward, frees the body completely as you become like a slippery fish setting itself free from a bullying

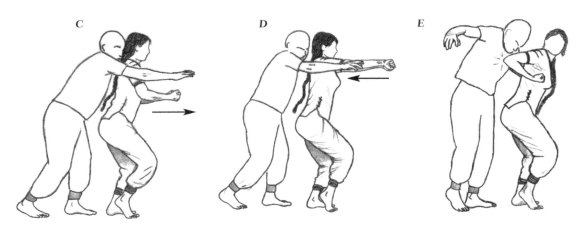

C   D   E

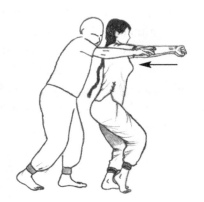 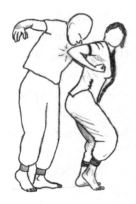

bear (or, better yet, a bullying human fisherman, for humans are the ones who best cultivate this quality). Finally, as always in life, sooner or later he who wants to be an abusive hunter winds up being hunted himself.

Keep present in your mind that the frontal projection is followed by only one backward projection of the elbows: either or both of them can easily reach their target.

Another application of this form of projection would be against two opponents: the one who has embraced you from behind and another in front of you, who would receive the full impact of the Force of the Double Spiral. This example is shown in the extra drawings, where you can see the student grabbed by two opponents. In the story told in the First Step, you may have noticed how Tara released herself from her attackers in this way; now it is your turn to make real what may sound like a legend!

> **Symbolic Name:** The Fish That Escapes
>
> **Initial Position:** Base Position
>
> **Steps Within the Movement:** 2 (3 seconds each)
>
> **Zone Taken:** Taken in a hug from behind, covering the arms
>
> **Technical and Respiratory Development (S=Step):** Base Position, two taps to the sides of your arms
>
>   S1. Bend your knees with the Force of the Double Spiral. Inhale (*nsss!*).
>
>   S2. Project both of your elbows behind you. Exhale (*haaa!*).
>
>   Osseous Field

31. Form of Reaction to Being Taken— Number 3: The Force of a Direct Reaction

We will now use our imagination again to learn a new form of reaction, but this time it will be in response to our being taken from the front, with our imaginary opponent facing us and taking the sides of both our upper arms with a firm grip. We will use a way similar to number 28, only this time against someone who is grabbing us. In this way you can easily value how one movement can have multiple functions, working from several different perspectives as a versatile and practical defense.

Development:

(A) From Osseous Field, indicate, with two small taps, one to each shoulder, where, in your imagination, you will be taken. With this, you are ready for the action.

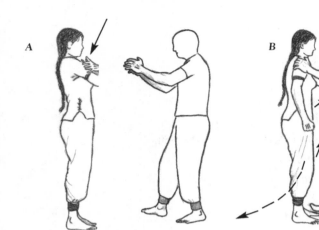

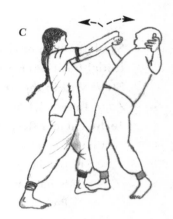

(B) *Action:* You are taken by your imaginary opponent from the front, firmly, on the sides of both of your shoulders.

(C) *Reaction:* Step back with your right foot in the Basic Step, and at the same time bring your fists to your sides (The Solid Fist) and execute the Crossed High Block (number 11). Do all of this in only one movement, inhaling and exhaling (*nsss! haaa!*).

(D) Immediately, our imaginary opponent must loosen his grip because of both the pressure of our forearms on his arms and the strike to his face, which has forced him back. Open your arms simply, both hands in fists, to clear the area in front and prevent any action. They need be no wider than your shoulders. Inhale (*nsss!*).

(E) Project The Whip Foot high, to the face of your imaginary opponent, exhaling (*haaa!*).

Then, return (right joining left) to the beginning, bringing your feet together and finishing in Osseous Field.

Just as in the previous form of reaction, our release in this situation has been formed by the union of various elements: the step; the arms as they ascend in the crossed block, which in this situation

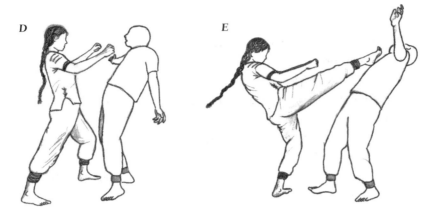

D   E

works also as a powerful strike that would easily neutralize a stronger opponent, forcing him back; and as if this were not enough, the projection of the leg, acting as a final element of extraordinary power. May this, which on first glance you can see as a form of defense, support your discovery of the factors that will help you to release your own mind: positivity, energy, dedication, creativity, and a *big* desire to learn and experience forever!

Symbolic Name: The Force of a Direct Reaction
Initial Position: Osseous Field
Steps Within the Movement: 3 (4 seconds)
Zone Taken: Both of your shoulders taken by two hands
Technical and Respiratory Development (S=Step):
Osseous Field, two taps to the sides of your shoulders
- S1. Go backward with your right foot in the Basic Step, combined in the same instant with the Crossed High Block. Inhale and exhale (*nsss! haaa!*).
- S2. Open your arms. Inhale (*nsss!*).
- S3. High Whip Foot with the right. Exhale (*haaa!*).
Osseous Field

With this, our last form of reaction, we have completed this stage. From here on, what is left is perfection, through a regular, meticulous practice. With time, you will be able to execute the entire sequence of Forms of Reaction continuously, one after the other, as you focus completely in coordinative continuity, imagination, and instinct. Think positive, for the Inner Power has always been there! You have already taken your second step now on the road to discovering it!

Stage VI. Meditation and Closing the Class

32. Breathing Technique of the Inner Power

After completing the previous cycle, always execute the Breathing Technique of the Inner Power twice; for details go to the Jass-U Stage (chapter 2, exercise 5). This is a simple way to recover your energy and to symbolically close each class or stage of teaching.

33. Final Meditation: Closing the Circle

Now sit down, as shown in the drawing, or in whatever way is more comfortable for you. Place your hands in front of you (as in the Breathing Technique of the Inner Power) and inhale deeply (A), contain (B), and exhale (C) as slowly as possible, closing your eyes. Place your arms on your legs as shown in the final drawing.

Rest for a while in this position (one or two full minutes), remaining as quiet and still as possible. In your mind, recall all the

A
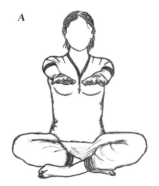

B
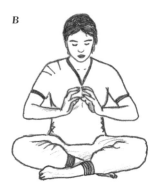

C
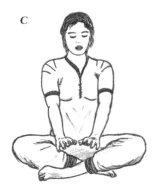

movements you have just executed, then review your whole class, seeing yourself doing the movements, full of energy and vitality, developing all of them easily, with agility and grace, as if you had known this Art from when you were a child. See yourself strong yet relaxed, willing and ready to face any storm! Keep this sensation of energy, and let it linger in your mind . . .

Meanwhile, your breathing must gently accompany you in the background, as a bellows that feeds the great inner flame, now keeping that flame ever burning inside you, in the center of your mind. The flame expands and contracts softly with the inhalation and exhalation, as if it were beating full of life.

Finally, see yourself surrounded by a protective aura, a mist that manifests itself like an egg of energy; this will prepare you to feed, or capture the positive, and at the same time it will protect you in the face of all the aggressiveness and negativity that may surround you. May this force teach you to think and decide for yourself!

Once you are finished, blink slowly and quietly stand up again.

Remember that every energy can be developed, and that this depends on you, just as does your self-cultivation and your overcoming of prejudices and negative energies, so that you may finally develop the potential that exists inside every human being, and therefore within you, too, as you transform yourself into a positive creative element, an element who can help both yourself and others.

Put your imagination to work and discover within Boabom the Great Inner Power! With this, relax and imagine that this sensation of force and life travels with you, completely: the Art and the energy that it generates over time will become one with you. May this new sensation be fruitful . . . and remember: think positive!

Congratulations! Congratulations! Congratulations!

and

May the Cosmic Winds always blow in your favor!

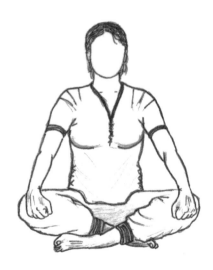

Chapter 5

The End and the Beginning of a Tale

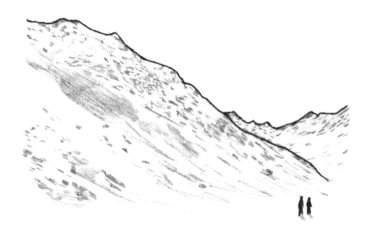

Life is the harvest of a short season,
which you must make the most of.

—*Seime, "The Knitter,"*
from The Legend of the Mmulmmat

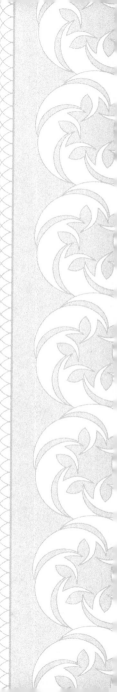

THE BONFIRE CONTINUED to burn strong. Then, after some time it began to die, with no one noticing; the students had been left lost in their own thoughts by the tale their Guide had told that night, too lost even to perceive that the flame was now turning into lonely coal. No one asked a single question, though all had many in their heads. Somehow the story had made them revive their own experiences and their deepest visions of the Art.

Slowly they began to understand that each movement, each coordination, each miniscule element of the Art had a special importance, an effect on their lives and on the lives of those who were able to take it into practice with enthusiasm and positive energy.

At last, the Guide arose quietly. Everyone else immediately woke from the silence of their thoughts. One group occupied themselves with extinguishing the fire, another brought a bit of order to the place; it was time now to rest. The death of the fire had made the light of the stars shine even stronger.

After a short while, all had left for their respective refuges. At the edge of the camp, only the Guide and his oldest student, he whom the Guide had named Black Sheep, remained.

Finally, the student asked a question. "What should the moral of your tale be?"

"Perhaps there is none . . . perhaps there is . . ." was the teacher's answer. "What do you think it should be?"

The young man stood, gazing at the stars that mantled the great dome. He did not know what to think, or maybe he had too many answers at the same time, all needing to be digested and analyzed. For this, he was unsure which would be the best moral to choose, and he remained silent for a moment. Finally, he dared to speak again.

"I think that the moral is that, even though Nnu-Suto took a risk by showing his teaching—" He continued, insecure—"it was worth it at last."

The Guide smiled and said, "I was not thinking that, but now that you mention it, do you really think that it was worth the risk of turning an entire town against him?"

"Well, he knew the risk he was taking and he made a decision," was the young man's reply.

"It is true. But he made a decision based on the fact that he would be in that place only for a short season. Whether the place was adequate or not would not affect him in the long term. But if he were to teach in that town for a long time, the risks would be different, both for him and for anyone who would listen—"

"But you have taught . . . and . . ."

The Guide completed the thought. "Mmm . . . and why could you not do the same someday? Is that what you wanted to say?"

"Well, not exactly."

"Seeing oneself is a difficult task, Black Sheep, and teaching others that point of view is almost impossible," said the Guide, who continued firmly. "It is not yet your time, for you are not prepared."

The Apprentice was silent, a bit embarrassed; only that morning they had been discussing the same subject.

THE END
AND THE
BEGINNING OF
A TALE

. . .

The Guide continued. "You still have much to learn of and overcome within yourself, much to discover of these teachings . . . then think about delivering them; if you do, the more complicated issue is to know who you are teaching and if this person will know how to value them. Yet what requires even more care is the fact that just as Boabom can be a double-edged sword, the teachings behind it can be so too." The young man looked in surprise at his Guide, who continued speaking. "What you see in one way, others can see in totally the opposite; what you understand as knowledge of one-self, others can see as an attack on their beliefs; what you feel are prejudices, others can feel as valuing their traditions and attach-ments; what you call evolution, in the interests of others can be seen as revolution; what you can express as the rectitude of free-dom, others who listen will take to mean a justification of their self-ishness and lack of humility. And what you naturally see as the consubstantial equality of all sensitive beings—be sure that will be seen as impracticable insanity and an offense to the greatness of man. In all times and all places you must walk with care—that is the experience of our teaching."

After a moment, the young man spoke again. "I understand. . . . You have explained that to me in many ways, and I suppose it is for that reason that your knowledge has been and remains for so few people," and then he added, with a tone of hope, "But couldn't it be more open?"

"Black Sheep, Black Sheep . . . human beings are unpredictable, contradictory. Most of them do not value, only treasure, do not learn, only imitate. It is very difficult finding the right person for this teach-ing, and it has always been so. Even if you do not want it to be so, it is difficult to make it in another way; besides, people like easy things, without commitments, things that let them quickly say that they have something, something that they can show off over others. Our Arts are invisible—who could boast of them? Besides, they are too complex and require time—*much* time—and when it is about cultivating yourself, no one has the time. It is considered foolish. The nature of our Art is not accessible."

"But it could be more accessible, right?"

"You keep insisting on being the Black Sheep. Could Nnu-Suto teach the entire town? No, only one person accompanied him until the end. Our waves of time do not always agree with those who surround us. You search for your way and let others be in peace. Just because you come from a different world, of towns and people, does not mean you need to open their eyes. They have not asked you to. They would misunderstand and twist it, criticize you mercilessly. As I have said before, every word that came from your mouth could have an evil meaning in their ears; your aspect would be improper, your way inadequate, and, lastly, your teaching would not belong to their time, to their culture. First prepare yourself."

"And how should I do that?"

"Seek . . . continue seeking. If you feel this Art, delve into it. It will carry you to the next steps that you must take."

The Apprentice asked immediately, "And what would the next steps be?"

"Patience," the Guide answered calmly and added, a bit mysterious, "you should pay more attention to the details of the tale, for perhaps the next step will not be only here. Perhaps it will be beyond the state of wakefulness."

The Apprentice was again thoughtful; he knew they were camping for just a few days. They would soon have to return to the city, to their own personal activities that would be happily interrupted only by their weekly classes in the Art. He did not want to miss this op-

THE END
AND THE
BEGINNING OF
A TALE
. . .

291

portunity to clarify his thoughts, for he felt that this was the most appropriate place to speak openly about the subject. There were few occasions such as this: only once a year did they organize a pilgrimage such as the one of this season, which included only the students who were closest to the Guide. Finally the Apprentice asked his question, trying to solve the puzzle. "But what do you mean? I would like to learn more . . . now." His Guide replied, avoiding a concrete answer, "Now? Now? Ah! Now it has been a great day and tomorrow will be an even greater one. Now go and rest, for a *great* dream awaits."

The Apprentice knew that there was no point in insisting: whenever his singular teacher began answering in this way, one had to leave the questions for another occasion. Maybe, as his Guide had said, it wasn't yet his time. He was aware that he had to advance more in Boabom and that the next year would be intense.

They respectfully said good-bye and each left for his own refuge. When the Apprentice had walked a few steps and his Guide was already some distance away, he was sure he could hear the Guide saying or singing something unintelligible. "Bamso . . . Bamso . . . Bamso . . ." The young man turned to see if the Guide was addressing him, but the Guide was already beyond his sight. Perhaps those words were only the whisperings of the wind in the mountains, or his imagination and nothing else.

It had truly been a long night. The dawn had awoken with the soft whispers of Seamm-Jasani; during the day there was much different work, typical of camping in the wilderness. The dusk then had belonged to the Osseous Art, Boabom.

Now it was the turn of the most mysterious of the Arts, the one that only whispered like a confused breeze past the ears of the Apprentice: "Bamso . . . Bamso . . . Bamso, the Art of Dreams," a path still far from his knowledge, a road that speaks the truth of oneself, even when that truth is too improper for our perspectives. But oh! Great Reality! Thank you for never adapting to anyone's mind! Thank you for happening free, as incomprehensible as ineffable! Elusive muse, invisible and certain, that without pity or hatred chases the self-centered mind of the thinkers, that undoes the ideas exhausted in themselves and disintegrates all faculty that lives in constant struggle with its ghosts.

There, in this last Art, the most sublime, the most fine of them all, Black Sheep was to transform his name and begin the search for the answers to his deepest questions.

Full Moon
Twenty-and-third day
Second month
Circle of the Sun of the Time of the Emenise
Land of the End of the World

THE END

AND THE

BEGINNING OF

A TALE

. . .

Third Step

THE SCHOOL

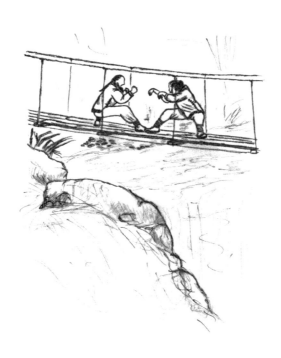

A Guide and an apprentice form a line of teaching,
but not necessarily a fruit.
Just as three apprentices form a school,
but not necessarily a fruit.
But it is enough if one of them values the teachings
and is capable of building with his hands
the ideas sowed in his mind
to find ourselves before a fruit.

—*from* The Memories of the Mmulargan

The Schools of Boabom

Its Stages, Principles, and Language

Now that you already know the foundations of the Art, it is time to delve into how Boabom and its schools are managed today. Just as I have mentioned before, this teaching develops a wide variety of evolutionary systems of movements, which are treated from different perspectives: one of them is Boabom, the Osseous Art, which you have just studied in the Second Step. But the method of the classes goes far beyond just this.

In general, the School has its own order; it develops a simple and universal Way to deliver this Art to its students. To bring this into practice, first it uses a singular language; second, it establishes essential principles that give it character and definition as a School; and third the pedagogy of the teachings is developed in branches, grades, and stages of learning.

As for this first aspect, the School has its own code language or mantric language that goes beyond national roots and through which the teacher can be technically understood by any other who teaches as she does and, on the other hand, can through this same language, transmit to her students the secrets and essential structure of the Art.

The word-sound is the first step in these ideas. Each movement has its own singular name, which is united to a specific concept. For a beginner this gives a sense of order to the movements, and for the advanced apprentice this code language speaks the history and background of each movement, its reach and profound goals. I have obviously not been able to use this language directly in this book, but I have indeed, as you may have noticed, created an approach and given symbolic names to the different movements that are developed in the Second Step. The idea is for this book to be as understandable, practical, and open as possible for students who are beginning or have no previous preparation whatsoever.

In respect to the second point, it is important to mention that, just as was said in chapter 8 of the First Step, the Schools of Boabom follow a Code of conduct that identifies their character and thought. In this sense, this Code recognizes the balance and unity that must exist between Body-Mind and Art, this last being the natural manifestation of the previous.

From this balance are born certain essential and practical ideas: discipline, respect, and humility, so that the student might learn to develop the Art fully, and at the same time can understand these ideas as advice for life that each, by her or his own measure and free will, must learn to carry into daily reality. To follow this advice one need belong neither to any specific religion nor to a certain race of special status; one need only have just a little human common sense, as exists in town or any place on this earth. Think that discipline, respect, and humility are necessary elements and that they must always be applied to any task from which we expect to have a result that is, in the end, positive.

Beginning from this base, the School seeks to develop the Art through its students and to transmit to them, with the highest possible fidelity, both the technique and the essential values that are born with it. Obviously, each teacher will always have a personality, individual criteria, and a level of exigency in order to deliver what she or he carries, but all of them must respect the principles that are the manifestation of the Code of the Art.

In daily and immediate practice, this Code, or Principle, is translated into three other, linked elements: first, the vision of the Art as a manifestation of the personal psychical work; second, nonviolence; and third, noncompetition. Thus, in Boabom as an Art of Internal Defense, you see that all of its movements are executed in imagination or focused in a meditative way. Respect among classmates becomes something natural, for the objective is the knowledge of oneself through movement. This is why in the School of Boabom one will never find the worshiped picture of a master from the past or present, for all guidance is only a bridge to look at yourself not a goal per se, as many Eastern teachings tend to misunderstand (and, by the way, Western teachings too!).

Following a chain of logical consequence, as students get to know themselves, they become emptied of fear and begin to develop self-control, confidence, and energy, and with this any attitude of violence or tendency toward it vanishes, bit by bit, like a handful of earth on which we pour spring water.

Finally, the schools that develop this Art are aware that it is *not* a sport and that therefore there is *no* space for trophies within them. Our idea of a School has no relation whatsoever to the concept of

Academy or Gym, where competition is part of the daily exercise; on the contrary, any kind of comparison among the students would never be encouraged or even allowed, and even less likely would be the possibility of any of them having the slightest inkling of participating in any kind of tournament. If this did happen, it would prove two things: that the person in question was never actually a Boabom student, or if he had been one, then he was a poor beginner who never understood anything about this teaching. Besides, life cannot be summarized in a championship! Or in a sales chart! I am aware that there are many people who will not like what I am about to write, so please excuse me ahead of time, but I must say it. Let's leave the winners and losers stuff to those who live obsessed with the sick modern society (sorry!)—just one more culture among the thousands of others that have been and will be!

Well, as usual I have gotten a little overenthusiastic in my writing. Let us continue with the development of the School, the subject that interests us. Coming now to the third point in our earlier description, I will show the path of growth that the Art must present in a fully-formed School. You will see that it has branches, grades, and stages.

Boabom itself represents one branch; Seamm-Jasani represents another, constituting one of the siblings of Boabom. In the book *The Secret Art of Seamm-Jasani,* I mentioned that this was only "the very tip of the iceberg"; this is so. As a hint at what lies beneath and at the same time as a way of explaining how the branches, degrees, and stages develop within this teaching, I have added a schematic diagram that explains the general evolution one should find in a School. The diagram outlines only a summary of the degrees and states in relation to Boabom, the Osseous Art, which is the central current of this book. This chart should give you an idea of what students can expect if they attend classes regularly.

Thus we have, from top to bottom (see illustration):

First State, the Fundamental School with:
Branches: Seamm-Jasani, Boabom, Art of Elements, etc. . . . .
General Boabom Stages: Lower and middle stages of the student's pedagogical development.
Degrees of Boabom: Different levels that the student covers within Boabom.
Technical Evolution of Boabom: Graphic volume of subjects developed in each level.
Technical Styles of Boabom: Concepts achieved in the different levels.

Second State, or the Higher School, and a Third State, or Internal School: A general idea of what these cover.
In Parallel, the ideas of *Mechanical Defense (External Movement), Spontaneous Defense, and Invisible Defense (Inner Power),* and how these take life and evolve within Boabom, through all the states of our School. This is directly related to what is discussed in chapter 6 of the story (First Step).

A fundamental School of Boabom is always under the direction of an independent but authorized teacher. Today there is a General Council, formed by senior teachers, who are in charge of the formation of new Assistants and Teachers.
In this outline are named some of the branches, as well as the eight basic stages of Boabom: each of these covers a style of movement that is completely different from the others, which means that what you study in the Second Stage is completely different from what you study in the First, and so on. The movements developed in

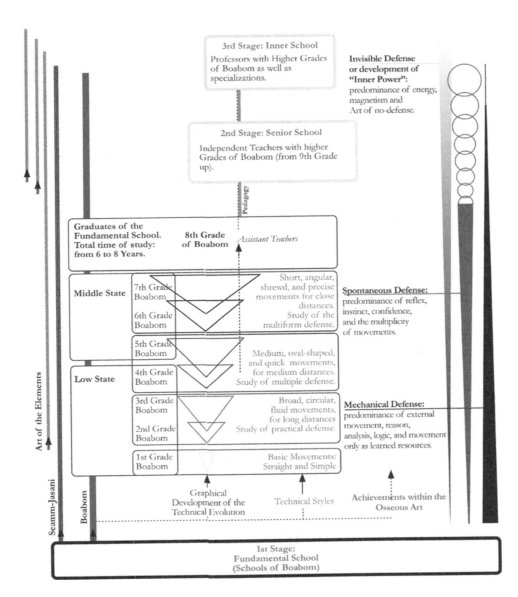

3rd Stage: Inner School

Professors with Higher Grades of Boabom as well as specializations.

Invisible Defense or development of "Inner Power": predominance of energy, magnetism and Art of no-defense.

2nd Stage: Senior School

Independent Teachers with higher Grades of Boabom (from 9th Grade up).

Pedagogy

Graduates of the Fundamental School. Total time of study: from 6 to 8 Years.

8th Grade of Boabom

Assistant Teachers

Middle State

7th Grade Boabom

6th Grade Boabom

Short, angular, shrewd, and precise movements for close distances. Study of the multiform defense.

Spontaneous Defense: predominance of reflex, instinct, confidence, and the multiplicity of movements.

5th Grade Boabom

4th Grade Boabom

Low State

Medium, oval-shaped, and quick movements, for medium distances. Study of multiple defense.

3rd Grade Boabom

2nd Grade Boabom

Broad, circular, fluid movements, for long distances. Study of practical defense.

Mechanical Defense: predominance of external movement, reason, analysis, logic, and movement only as learned resources.

1st Grade Boabom

Basic Movements: Straight and Simple

Graphical Development of the Technical Evolution

Technical Styles

Achievements within the Osseous Art

Art of the Elements

Seamm-Jasani

Boabom

1st Stage: Fundamental School (Schools of Boabom)

Diagram of the complete School

this book constitute about five percent of the movements of only the First Stage! I would have to write at least twenty books like this one to even superficially develop the first of these eight levels, only the tip of the iceberg! And remember too that I am speaking only of Boabom, for I have not referred in detail to Seamm-Jasani, or other branches, such as the Art of Elements, or higher forms of Meditation, since all of them have an independent development that is equally profound.

These ideas are only an example of why we call Boabom the Art of a Thousand Ways. In truth, the School is comprised of many more than one thousand ways.

Yesterday, Today, and Tomorrow

Currently, the only real evidence of this teaching is its students, the heirs of Boabom. The stories of this Art speak of a mythical time, taking this tradition back more than ten thousand years, into the vast region that would someday be known as Tibet. The legends are many, and it would be worth unfolding them in one or many books, but for now I will only say that it is said that since that immemorial time, Guides and Apprentices have given life to Boabom and its Way in the subtle silence of far mountains or forgotten villages. I cannot, however, certify or prove precisely the exact time and place; I can only transmit the certainty given in the oral teachings I have received, as well as the ancient stories that indicate that all the Eastern and Western traditions come from only one root.

On one side, the true antiquity of this Art cannot be proven by carbon-14 dating, or something of that sort, but on the other, it can be proven by feeling its effects in the daily lives of those who have immersed themselves in this teaching. This is the best of all, the most real, tangible, and useful for those who live in this era or in any time; thus nowadays we can have evidence of the value and profundity of these teachings, which is within the grasp of anyone who wishes to look for it with discipline and constancy, and is capable of living it with positive energy.

There is still much to tell, so let us leave these inquietudes for the future and for the right ears. The most important thing is that today a new generation of Teachers has already been born, who have the transmission of Boabom under their responsibility. Whether in the silence of the mountains or inside a studio located in the heart of a great, active city, this Art, in all its forms, is expanding its life day after day.

In the next chapter it will be the students' turn; they are the living School. The students are the blood of the body of this teaching, and as such they had to put their seal on this book too; we have included the testimonies of a wide range of students. Some of them are student-readers who have followed the book *The Secret Art of Seamm-Jasani* and have sent us their comments via e-mail, remarking on all the positive effects they have seen; others have traveled continents, only their books under their arms, seeking to develop and deepen themselves in the knowledge of this Art in all its aspects. There are also beginning and advanced students from the Boabom Schools of various countries, all of whom wished to be present in this summary of comments: they represent a new generation of the Boabom Arts in all of their forms, and it must be they who speak the benefits of this Art on their lives. I hope that the diversity in their points of view presented here will be useful to you as you come to understand this teaching.

In the final stage of this book, a group of professionals, with the collaboration of some of our Teachers, have taken it upon themselves to research and create an investigative study with all the rigors of modern science. In regard to this work, I would like to recognize our senior and dedicated Teacher Mobanie, for all of her energy and will in accomplishing this project, as well as the psychologist Francisco D. Göpfert and Dr. Ismael Carvajal for their discipline and professional rigor in the design, evaluation, and delivery of the final report.

They have completed the first study ever made about this Art based on scientific criteria. The results speak for themselves . . . now it is you who must try this reality.

When the Students Speak

"Although all legitimate martial arts schools hope to improve the health and security of their students, from my personal experience with many teachings, I feel that Boabom offers something completely unique. The simplest way to express this is to say that I actually feel healthier, more energetic, and *happier* after each class.

"As a physician, I know people need to breathe and move in healthy ways to maximize their functions. How wonderful to find a well-developed and time-tested system of movements that create this health, a sense of joy, and the ability to protect oneself while the student is actually relaxing throughout the class!"

—Lawrence Wolfe, M.D.
Associate professor, Department of Pediatrics
Tufts University School of Medicine
North Grafton, Massachusetts

Seamm-Jasani and Boabom Training Experience and Reflections

"It was only when I began the practice of Seamm-Jasani and Boabom that I finally understood the real significance of the chakra. I began with Seamm-Jasani, buying the book out of simple curiosity. It was 'yet another system' to explore for me. Frankly, having seen similarities in philosophy and details among so many 'different' methods and styles, I didn't actually expect to harvest anything truly novel. But I began the practice with my usual exploratory spirit.

Right away, within the first hour of my first self-training session, guided only by the first Seamm-Jasani book, I felt a harmonizing and smoothing of my energy field and body that I had never before experienced. It was a supremely soothing effect of gentle calming. From that first experience, my internal 'ears' perked up, and I realized there must be a lot more to this system than is apparent from a superficial glance.

"That night I had the most profound energetic-spiritual experience of my entire life, directly triggered by that evening's Boabom class. I can't describe what happened when I lay down to sleep after that first class any better than to say that my solar-plexus center burst open for the first time. The words may be flowery, but the experience was absolutely, blissfully annihilating. It seemed that a huge high-voltage electric plug had been extended directly from the center of the universe and precisely custom-fit to an electric socket located exactly at my solar-plexus center. I realized that this effect had been consciously created by the Boabom system. Boabom, undergirded by the physical and spiritual preparation of the Seamm-Jasani preliminaries, is a coded, non-obvious work of ancient genius. You could say it is a form of ancient secret 'technology'—a fantastically sophisticated technology of safe access to the very highest voltages of the universal energies. I now see that every single apparently small or insignificant or decorative posture, movement, alignment, or practice mode of Boabom is in fact a crucial integrated element in an unspeakably effective discipline of energetic reconnection to the Source.

"And what I particularly love about the Mmulargan school's teachings is that they haven't been used to create a cult, a religion, a belief system, or any other rigid orthodoxy. Rather than pushing doctrine and belief, the Mmulargan school emphasizes a gently nonverbal kind of direct experience that can be integrated into every individual student's life and value system entirely as he or she wishes. The unspoken message seems to be: believe anything you want. Just train and experience the simple 'reconnection.'"

—Scott Meredith, Ph.D.
Senior researcher, theoretical and
computational linguistics
Washington

"This Art, which has accompanied me since my childhood, can be seen from various perspectives: as a physical activity, but not just any physical activity—one which is extremely complex, at the same time easy and possible for all different kinds of people, drastically improving any deficiency in their motor capacity, giving them precision and strength, since it works with all the different groups of muscles (and really, with all of them!). It can also be seen as a system of defense, but when defense is mentioned in this Art, it is from a totally unique perspective. Boabom is totally effective, precise, nonroutine, and besides all this, it gives you confidence in every action in your life, whatever it may be. When it comes to health, we can see an improvement in condition across different types of ailments. I have seen and experienced this personally: from simple digestive problems and ulcers to chronic asthma and more. Another astonishing element I have seen is how sedentary people quickly recover their natural energy, sharpen their senses, increase their physical elasticity, and in general rejuvenate themselves.

"Boabom is a system that allows you to 'be' for the first time, meaning to think, for the first time, without reference to another (or without needing to compare yourself); at the same time, you over-come those barriers that society constantly forces on us, like preju-dice, competition, mockery, and the like. This Teaching is a path to individual perfection—and Art.

"This vision represents a brief sample of someone who has stud-ied this teaching since near the beginning of his existence, and has taken it primarily as a way of life and a continuous apprenticeship, being a fundamental foundation for everything I do and face in this odyssey we call life.

"From a faithful student and apprentice-Teacher of Boabom."

—Saulo Díaz
Medical student
Universidade Federal do Rio de Janeiro, Brazil

"I have spent much time in my life on sports, health, and body-mind practices—e.g., yoga for thirteen years. Last year I came across a book about this Art. I tried the exercises and—unlike some other books I bought in the past—I actually found these exercises great! The book was clear and to the point. After more practice I got more enthusias-tic and looked up the website of this Art. I then decided to go to Boston in the United States to join an upcoming seminar, and I did several extra classes. I learned more and thoroughly enjoyed it. I now practice regularly at home. This is a great way to health! The Art is easily accessible, and you'll notice straightaway how it energizes your body. I've particularly found the combination of moving and breath-ing in this Art excellent. It completely involves all your attention. I can notice how much more grounded and centered I have become in my body. And what's more, it is fun to do these exercises. And that keeps you doing them."

Donatus Roobeek

Manager of health clinic, swimming and yoga teacher

UK

"It is difficult to express in a few words how important knowing Boabom has been to me, in all its forms, as an art of relaxation and defense. The development of both physical and mental skills has been astonishing, specifically useful and noteworthy to me as a businessman with a demanding and stressful schedule. I think that Boabom is key to the success of all people who wish to have control over their own lives, and at the same time who are looking to complete their ideas with the energy and vitality required these days."

Marcelo Robles

International businessman

Chile

"I enjoyed Seamm-Jasani class very much, and my teacher is great and fun. I have always enjoyed high energy and creativity in this class. It helped me to achieve body equilibrium and restoration. My teacher's explanations are always clear, and the atmosphere at the lessons is very enjoyable. The most important part of this program for me is to pay attention to posture. I learned how to achieve effortless balance without strain. I have problems with my cervical muscles and disks, and Seamm-Jasani is the only training where I feel no pain after the lessons. I think the secret is in its unique breathing pattern. Seamm-Jasani is an easy-to-follow, ancient Art that anyone can do."

Lucy Aronova
Piano teacher
U.S.A.

"Throughout the ages, the relationship between the physical and the mental has been a matter of debate. In the Boabom philosophy, such a relationship is prominently present. However, even if this assumed relationship would not exist at all, Boabom leads to various absolute physical improvements.

"Unlike many other sports, Boabom also appeals to the elderly, a group not prone to exercise. By improving your balance, forces applied to joints are ameliorated, thus relieving strain and wear on them. It can thus greatly reduce long-term lower-back and joint pain. Also improved balance reduces risk of falling, which is a great source of mortality and morbidity among the elderly.

"It keeps you in shape, so you will perform better in daily life. And of course one could argue it is also fun!"

Paul Jeene
Medical student
Netherlands

"I feel more positive in my approach to my everyday life now—more awake, more clearheaded. Physically, I feel better than I have in a long time. I feel strong, flexible, and more relaxed. I feel happier, healthier (they do go hand in hand). Physical problems that were nagging before have diminished noticeably or disappeared. My focus and confidence in general are greatly improved, and I feel I am becoming more in tune with what I need in my life internally and externally and what I do not. Soon after I began the class, I felt a positive effect quickly. Since, this effect has continued to grow in surprising ways. It began with self-defense and became so much more. I feel a great deal of gratitude for everything Boabom has helped to awaken within me."

Jennifer Winslow
Technical writer
U.S.A.

"Like all natural things, everything has a beginning and a development. For me, arriving at the School a few years ago has meant an awakening from a long and profound lethargy. Just like a tiny sprout, with the passage of time I have grown into the teachings of this Art, and have cultivated a steely discipline which has meant a better and stronger life. I have eradicated small vices, such as smoking and a generally sedentary life. I can also affirm a dramatic improvement in my mobility, resistance to stress, muscular agility, breathing capacity, and especially in knowing how to observe, assay, and measure any adversary—any problem in general—without fear, achieving confidence in myself and my actions."

Juvenal Buccarey
Naval officer, retired
Second-in-Command of Antarctic Mission (1977–1979),
Arturo Prat Naval Base, Chile

"Although Boabom is an ancient Art, I feel that, in these days of cubicles, computers, and automobiles, it is needed more than ever for its wellspring of personal health and wellness."

Stephen Fell
Musician and teacher
U.S.A.

"The Art has been a great discovery for me. I have never been so comfortable with any discipline, never so confident and so happy practicing it. I do not drown in a glass of water anymore, and when faced with anything I breathe, as in my classes, I become calm— and then the answer comes."

Joan Hudson
Businesswoman
Chile

"From the perspective of Traditional Chinese Medicine, Boabom is unique in that it helps people find balance both within their bodies and in the way they engage and interact with the world, no matter what their particular background, lifestyle, personality, stress level, or fitness level may be. Many Eastern arts like yoga and tai chi, while they may be extremely beneficial in helping people cultivate their yin energy (balance, flexibility, breathing, and relaxation), are less focused on developing yang energy (power, speed, quick reactions, assertiveness). The reverse is true of many of the Eastern martial arts that focus on developing yang energy, which they do through a lot of strength and speed training, as well as through contact, sparring, and breaking exercises, while not focusing on the development of yin energy.

"Boabom is as beneficial to a person with a predominantly yin constitution as it is to a person with a predominantly yang constitution. I have always been somewhat of a shy person, and my experiences with Boabom have been invaluable in teaching me how to unfold and develop my yang energy and have helped me with self-confidence and assertiveness. I have no doubt that if necessary I could react and defend myself in a threatening situation. For yang-type individuals—people with high energy or stress levels, who are naturally more extroverted and easily aggravated—Boabom helps them to connect with their yin energy through its focus on breathing and meditation in order to help them achieve relaxation, self-control, and balance. In my experience, Boabom has a unique approach that differs from other Eastern Arts because it helps individuals cultivate internal and external balance through the development of both their yin and yang energy."

Heather Lance
B.A. in Asian studies
Graduate student in acupuncture and Oriental medicine

"As I went through the movements that make up the first two stages of Boabom, I was struck by how much better my balance, coordination, flexibility, strength, and endurance have become over the past years and even recent months. What is more intriguing to me, however, and much more difficult to explain, are the mental changes that have come as a result of studying the Art. It is not so much that I'm more relaxed, though I believe that I am, but rather that I am more mentally alert and agile. The challenges in Boabom are both physical and mental, and that is what makes it such a rewarding art to study. I look forward to the challenges that lie ahead in future stages!"

Susanna Bolle
Writer, music critic, and DJ
U.S.A.

"Most people realize that they need to exercise, that daily life is too fast paced and stressful, that they need to slow down and celebrate life. Yet all these things are quite difficult to do on your own, particularly when you don't know 'how' to relax, to move with grace and balance, to celebrate your body and spirit. As I've practiced and reflected on what I've learned over the last three-plus years studying Boabom, I've realized that here is a friendly, structured art that does all these things. Only a few years ago, simple things I now take for granted—like balancing on one foot, breathing deeply during intense exercise, and engaging in coordinated movements that initially 'teased' my brain—were a struggle. Yet my muscles and joints have grown stronger, my sense of balance has improved, my brain can better direct 'right' and 'left' movements. Even as I've experienced some illnesses that slowed my progress over the last year, the Art has accommodated me and allowed me to progress, and in the process it has certainly contributed positively to my health and well-being. As I prepare to move to a new stage, I am just now beginning to really sense that Boabom is more than a series of physical and mental challenges, and I look forward to experiencing greater spiritual well-being through these practiced movements and relaxation techniques."

Shaun Gummere
Director of Web services and professor of Web design
U.S.A.

"Practicing Boabom is the best thing that has ever happened to me. Being happy in life causes those who surround you to be infected with that optimism; joy has a multiplying effect. This is achieved when you are in harmony with your mind and body, and that is the objective of this Art."

Ana María Gómez
Bilingual secretary
Chile

Visit this website for more student comments:
http:www.asanaro.com/comments

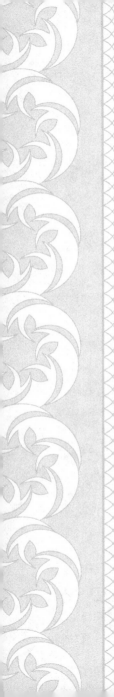

A First Scientific Approach to the Boabom Arts*

Francisco D. Göpfert, Psychologist
Ismael Carvajal González, M.D.

Introduction

The influence of air and breathing on the development of the human beings is not yet a completely understood process, and that goes beyond the purely physiologic ambit. From the mother's womb, air is a vital element for the development of the fetus, which it receives through the placenta; this reflects its unity with and dependence on the mother. With the first breaths, as with physical separation through the cutting of the umbilical cord, the first movement of individuation is accomplished, the starting point of each new life, whose rhythm begins to be commanded by, among other things, breathing.

The ancient Greeks used the word *pneuma* to identify the concepts of air and soul, and they supposed that the first breath of the newborn was accompanied by the incorporation of the soul into the body, thus giving life, and that the exhalation of the last sigh of the dying meant the leaving of the soul and the death of the physical body.

Breathing, the process whose mechanical part we are so accustomed to that we do not even notice, can also, through the voluntary control of the implied muscles, be transformed into a conscious action.

*Descriptive exploratory study of the influence of Boabom arts on students, February 2005.

In the East, especially in Tibet, India, China, and Japan, there are ancient techniques of meditation, practiced by monks, based upon breathing; the benefits of these practices in the mental ambit is widely known. The constant and regular practice of any physical activity brings benefits in the physiological area, especially in the cardiopulmonary system, all of which are widely studied. However, what has not been studied is the influence on the human being of techniques that combine the meditation and the physical exercise, which could be called meditation in movement.

Boabom is a system of practice of diverse movements, coordinative and accumulative, associated with different types of breathing. Because of these characteristics, it seems relevant to study the influence of this practice on the physical and mental development of its students.

Methodology

A survey was made of the students of the Mmulargan School to evaluate the influence of the practice of Boabom, focusing on perception in the areas of physiology, physical development, sleep, and dreaming, with the goal of having a first exploratory descriptive approximation of the influence of this discipline in these aspects.

Instrument

A survey was made in which we asked: Since you have practiced Boabom, do you think you have experienced any change in the following aspects? For this, 27 indicators were enumerated, for each of which four answer choices were presented: yes, no, no variation, I do not understand the question.

These indicators were grouped in four categories:

1. Mental and psychological aspects
2. Physical aspects
3. Sleeping and dreaming and
4. Diseases and consumption of medication*

The instrument was submitted to the judgment of experts in order to evaluate their internal validity, and the pilot test was then applied to ten volunteers to evaluate the clarity of the indicators. These volunteers were not considered in the sample.

Sample

The sample comprised eighty-one regular students of various Boabom schools who voluntarily agreed to answer this survey. This voluntary acceptance was the only criterion used to define the investigated sample.

Procedure

Each student who volunteered to participate in this investigation was given a written survey, which she/he had to answer in private; the surveyors did not answer any explanatory questions and

*This aspect of the study provided inconclusive data. See "Limitations and Proposals of the Investigation," page 331.

limited themselves to indicating to the participating students only that they should carefully read the instructions and the document, trying thereby to avoid the inducement of any kind of bias from the surveyor to the participant.

Results

Presented here are the results, which for the investigators represent a greater meaning because of their implication as indicators and for their contribution to future investigations. Of the twenty-seven indicators, only thirteen were used, because the rest gave incomplete or nonsignificant data, totally excluding the dimension of diseases and substance consumption.

Mental and Psychological Aspects

1. Confidence in one-self (confidence in one's capacities)

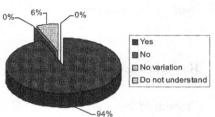

As can be seen in the graphic, 94 percent of the people surveyed indicated that the practice of Boabom had increased their confidence in their own capacities, a fundamental element for the strengthening of self-esteem and personal self-image.

The other 6 percent signaled that they kept the same confidence in their own capacities; it had not been modified by practicing the studied discipline.

2. Serenity in daily life

Eighty-two percent indicated that since initiating Boabom they had experienced a change in the serenity of their daily lives, which can imply the

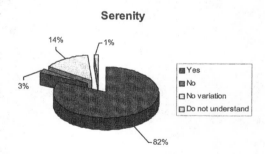

development of a personal skill that could favor the resolution of diverse relational conflicts.

3. Joy in daily activities

Of the 81 surveyed, 84 percent said that practicing Boabom had affected their emotional state positively, especially in the joy they had in their daily activities, which would probably influence their thoughts and projections for the future.

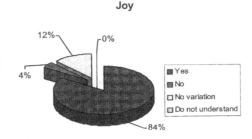

Joy

12% · 0%
4%
- Yes
- No
- No variation
- Do not understand
84%

4. Optimism (positive thoughts about future projections)

In findings very closely linked to those of the previous graphic, 88 percent of those surveyed answered that they have had an increase in positive thoughts of what might happen to them in the future. This likely indicates a positive outlook.

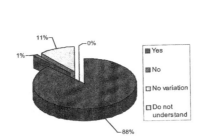

Optimism

11% · 0%
1%
- Yes
- No
- No variation
- Do not understand
88%

5. Perseverance in daily duties

Seventy-six percent of those interviewed said that Boabom had been influential in their daily perseverance. Probably, and given the previous indicators, the students could feel less frustrated when faced with

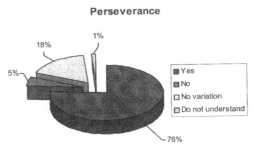

Perseverance

1%
18%
5%
- Yes
- No
- No variation
- Do not understand
76%

situations that once bothered them, and thus they could achieve their proposed objectives much more easily.

6. Concentration
Seventy-eight percent of the participating group indicated that the practice of Boabom had influenced their capacity to concentrate their attention, which can imply, among other things, quickly focusing on the problem that has to be solved. This capacity caused them to be less affected by external stimuli that might otherwise influence resolution of the task at hand.

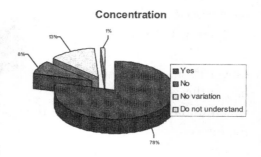

Concentration

- Yes
- No
- No variation
- Do not understand

13% 1% 8% 78%

Analysis of Mental and Psychological Aspects

Self-esteem, defined as "a feeling of acceptance and pride in oneself, combined with confidence in your own merit as an individual" would be indicated, among other ways, by the confidence one might have in one's capacities and by how much one is willing to count on oneself in the face of the different opportunities and options given us by daily life. The results obtained indicate that those who practice Boabom recognize the influence that it has had on their confidence and personal trust, happiness, optimism, perseverance, and concentration—all characteristics that contribute to a strengthening of self-esteem and a promotion of personal development. We must make clear that these variables have a personal connotation that the instrument used does not let us measure.

Physical Aspects

1. Decrease in physical tiredness

Ninety-five percent of those surveyed show an improvement in their muscular resistance, manifested by the decrease of physical tiredness in their daily activities.

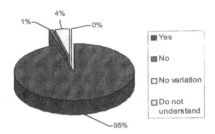

Resistance

2. Muscular elasticity

Ninety-nine percent of those surveyed refer to an improvement in their muscular elasticity, which is reflected in their reflexes and general agility.

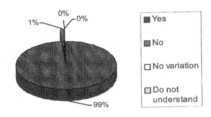

Elasticity

3. Breathing capacity

Ninety-five percent of those surveyed answered that they have had an improvement in their breathing capacity. It would be interesting, in future studies, to take objective measures of the breathing capacity through a manual peak-flow meter, especially in people who have asthmatic symptoms or any other respiratory conditions.

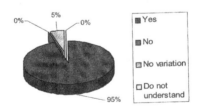

Respiratory Capacity

Analysis of Physical Aspects

The three aspects considered—muscular resistance, elasticity, and respiratory capacity—show the strong impact in the organism of the aerobic capacity developed by the practice of Boabom. The predominance in the use of the aerobic musculature over the anaerobic in this practice results in all the known benefits over the cardiopulmonary and vascular systems, such as: decrease of coronary disease and of atherosclerosis in major blood vessels, as well as the beneficial effect of the prevention of known risk factors for these diseases, such as obesity and the risk of diabetes mellitus associated with it.

Sleeping and Dreaming

In this category, the analysis was made by comparing two groups of fourteen students each, dividing the groups on the basis of the time they have practiced Boabom. To Group 1 belong students with four or more years, while in Group 2 are the students with three to eight months of practice.

In terms of indicators, the presence of premonitory dreams was also considered in a third group, which included the rest of those interviewed, who have practiced Boabom between eight months and four years.

1. Refreshing sleep

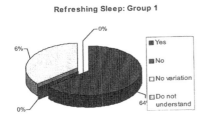
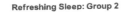
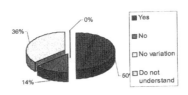

As for this question, we can see a slight difference between the two groups, where the most refreshing sleep is achieved by Group 1: the senior students.

2. Increase in length of dreams

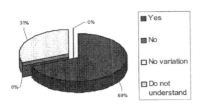
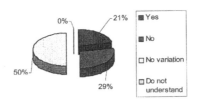

With this question we wished to explore the perception of the duration of each dream and to determine if the students noticed that their dreams had some kind of plot or progression. A great difference can be observed between the two groups: 69 percent of Group 1 shows an increase in the length of their dreams in comparison to only 21 percent of Group 2. This great difference serves as a basis for future investigations on this subject.

3.   Presence of dreams related to Boabom

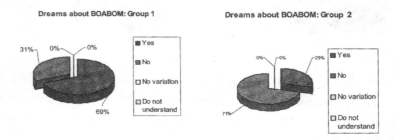

Dreams about BOABOM: Group 1

Dreams about BOABOM: Group 2

In this question, as in the previous one, we can also see a great difference between the two groups. While 69 percent of the senior students acknowledge dreaming about the activity of Boabom, only 29 percent of the junior students refer to dreaming of the discipline, a fact that calls our attention to the influence of the practice of this system on the students' dreams over time. This point also opens possibilities for future explorations.

4.   Premonitory dreams

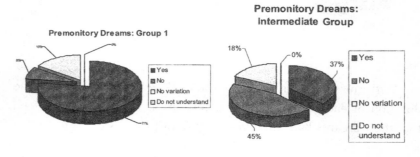

Premonitory Dreams: Group 1

Premonitory Dreams: Intermediate Group

In this question the exploration was made into events that were dreamed and then were experienced later on. One can appreciate a possible direct correlation between the time of practice and the presence of premonitory dreams. Seventy-seven percent of the senior group acknowledged having premonitory dreams, as compared with 37 percent of the intermediate group, and only 14 percent of the group with the least time of practice. This observation opens a wide range of investigable hypotheses, which range from the simple material influence on the level of the brain, to hyperventilation and state of concentration (necessary for the execution of the movements), to the intangible influence on those surveyed of the development within them, through the time in which they have practiced, of the values that Boabom proposes: discipline, respect, and humility.

Discussion

The investigation had as its objectives the organization, in a systematic way, of the informal comments of the benefits perceived by those who practice the discipline of Boabom, and the development of a first attempt at a scientific approximation of a descriptive, exploratory character, of the subjective implications perceived by the students in the psychological, physical, and oneiric ambits.

The study showed high percentages of positive answers in the psychological and physical dimension; the perception of an improvement in these areas could imply changes of higher importance for the interviewed, which are not yet evaluated and could be an important source of information for future investigations. Knowing that the sample chosen binds people of different ages, characters, personalities, cultures, and experiences of life, probably the personal meaning of the affirmation differs much from one to another of the interviewed, and therefore implicitly speaks more about harmonization than anything else, understanding as such the equilibrium between such poles as: aggressiveness-passivity (confidence in oneself), optimism-pessimism (joy and optimism), will and apathy (perseverance and concentration). For example, if we consider the pair aggressiveness-passivity, it is probable that the most aggressive person might have diminished such conduct in his daily life, presenting a higher control over himself, while on the other hand the timid person could be showing a higher force and confidence in the face of situations that used to cause anguish and fear. Another example could be given in the optimism/pessimism duet, where those with an excessive overvaluation of their own capacities could discover, through the practice of the exercises, their own limitations and learn from them, while those who tend to see the negative side could, through the progress obtained, begin to enjoy the sensation of optimism. On the other hand, the responses of improvement in the physical domain support the subjective sensations of psychical well-being. The improvement in muscular resistance to tiredness, in elasticity and agility of movement, and in respiratory capacity are by themselves indicators associated with a vital plenitude. It would be interesting for future investigations to relate these sensations to biological indicators or to morbid, acute, and chronic events in the lives of the practitioners of Boabom, knowing that the sensation of physical-psychical plenitude is associated with a more healthy and disease-free existence.

Within the category of sleeping and dreaming, the analysis of the results shows us a small difference in the physiological aspect of sleeping; it is in the aspect of dreaming, however, that we can appreciate the greatest influence of different lengths of time spent practicing, especially on the length and type of dreams. In the length of dreams indicator, as well as in the indicators of dreams related to Boabom, and especially in the premonitory dreams indicator, we find a stronger influence of the practice of this discipline on the development of a different quality of dreams. The percentages obtained allow us to conjecture that the influence of Boabom would be limited to the aspects manifested not only during wakefulness but also during the state of sleep.

Limitations and Proposals of the Investigation

Within the principal limitations recognized in the present investigation, the following can be indicated:

The instrument used:

1. Kind of Instrument: The survey as a way to obtain information does not allow access to data of a qualitative nature, which could be of great importance in understanding in greater depth the diverse effects of Boabom.
2. Construction of the instrument: The way in which the questions were asked in respect to diseases and consumption of medication, tobacco, and other things did not yield data clear enough to analyze; from this it seems necessary, if desiring to reapply the investigation, to modify the questions and the answer choices within this category.
3. Selection of the sample: By not discriminating based on variables such as gender, age, nationality, and previous state of

health, it was not possible to study and compare subpopulations.

The suggestions for future investigations are:

— A qualitative investigation that would allow for an analysis of oral answers delivered by the participants.

— A prospective investigation in which it is possible to compare the changes experienced by the same subject over time, from the beginning of the practice.

— Incorporate objective measures of breathing function, previous state of health, medication or tobacco consumption, and psychological aspects.

Final Comments

The results of the present investigation allowed us to make a first approach to the positive effects that for years were verbally described by those who practice the discipline of Boabom. Starting from the obtained results, as in any investigation new questions arise that can be answered only through future investigative efforts, whether along the proposed lines or in any new direction that might emerge from the creative mind of any reader. Despite this, we cannot forget that scientific thought is only one great method to come closer to knowledge, and in no way is it possible to fully broach the challenge of the individual experience. No matter how much we try to measure effects, understand processes, or evaluate the development of the practice of this discipline, no matter how much we analyze it in detail and later categorize the results, never will the whole be equal to the sum of the parts, and hardly will it be possible to transmit on paper the sensations and emotions of those who practice relaxation in movement, which, according to what has been presented in this work, gives multiple benefits to human development and to the quality of life of those who practice it. Investigation is necessary: it allows us to organize and present to others something as positive as Boabom, but it is naïve to think that it is enough.

About the Authors of This Study

Francisco D. Göpfert is a psychologist who has developed his career working in four fields. He has worked with at-risk populations, specifically those who have broken the law and are mentally challenged. He has taught psychology at the undergraduate level, and has done consulting work in organizational development, implementing programs to improve the quality of human capital in various organizations. He has also worked in private consultation with families and teenagers.

Ismael Carvajal González, M.D., has practiced medicine since 1986. He obtained his specialization in homeopathic medicine in 1995, and since then has focused on clinical work in private practice, where he has achieved significant results in the treatment of diverse medical pathologies.

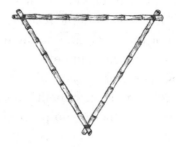

FURTHER INFORMATION

ASANARO, author of this book and teacher of the Arts described within, instructs at and supervises the Mmulargan School, a center for the Boabom Arts. These Arts are grounded in the understanding that body and mind form a perfect unity, essential and complete.

Within the Mmulargan School, three basic Arts are taught:

— Seamm-Jasani, or the Art for Eternal Youth, which is developed through fluid movements, meditation, and relaxation.

— Traditional Boabom, or the Osseous Art of defense and meditation of the Inner Path.

— Yaanbao, or the Art of Elements, which develops a complete cycle of coordinations, defense, and relaxation by using elements of various sizes and shapes as an extension of the movement.

For further information about the Mmulargan School, visit:

www.boabom.org
e-mail: boabom@boabom.org

Currently, the principal Boabom School in the United States is located in Boston. It offers regular classes through the primary development of these Arts, as well as special seminars and intensive courses. For more information on the Boston School of Boabom, please visit: www.bostonboabom.com.

Regarding authorized teachers: If you wish to contact a teacher who has been authorized by the School, or if you wish to know if your teacher has been certified, feel free to e-mail boabom@boabom.org.

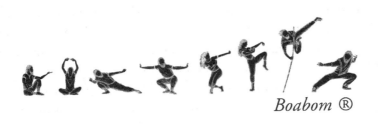

Boabom ®

ABOUT THE AUTHOR

Asanaro has dedicated more than twenty-five years to the study and transmission of the Boabom Arts, a path whose roots originated in pre-Buddhist Tibet. The teachings that Boabom is based on are transmitted in various ways, which cover breathing techniques, relaxation, defense, meditation, and philosophy.

Asanaro has taught around the world, offering courses, workshops, and seminars, and developing Boabom Schools in South America, Europe, and the United States. He has also been instrumental in the founding of many centers and associations for alternative arts and medicine.

He is the author of *The Secret Art of Seamm-Jasani: 58 Movements for Eternal Youth from Ancient Tibet,* a practical course-book; *Bamso: the Art of Dreams,* a metaphorical autobiographical story, which is also a guide to meditation and astral projection; and *The Legend of the Mmulmmat,* a book that tells the story of a lost world in the ancient mountains of Tibet (the Valley of the Warm Breeze) and describes the mythical origins of the Boabom teachings.

For more information about Asanaro, visit: http:www.asanaro.com.

If you wish to contact the author, ask questions, or make any comments, e-mail him at: asanaro@boabom.org.

. . .

Printed in the United States
by Baker & Taylor Publisher Services